CHILD WELFARE

CURRENT ISSUES, PRACTICES AND CHALLENGES

CHILDREN'S ISSUES, LAWS AND PROGRAMS

Additional books in this series can be found on Nova's website
under the Series tab.

Additional e-books in this series can be found on Nova's website
under the e-book tab.

SOCIAL ISSUES, JUSTICE AND STATUS

Additional books in this series can be found on Nova's website
under the Series tab.

Additional e-books in this series can be found on Nova's website
under the e-book tab.

CHILD WELFARE

CURRENT ISSUES, PRACTICES AND CHALLENGES

ALEX POWELL

AND

JENNA GRAY-PETERSON

EDITORS

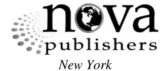

nova
publishers

New York

For permission to use material from this book please contact us:
Telephone 631-231-7269; Fax 631-231-8175
Web Site: http://www.novapublishers.com

NOTICE TO THE READER

The Publisher has taken reasonable care in the preparation of this book, but makes no expressed or implied warranty of any kind and assumes no responsibility for any errors or omissions. No liability is assumed for incidental or consequential damages in connection with or arising out of information contained in this book. The Publisher shall not be liable for any special, consequential, or exemplary damages resulting, in whole or in part, from the readers' use of, or reliance upon, this material. Any parts of this book based on government reports are so indicated and copyright is claimed for those parts to the extent applicable to compilations of such works.

Independent verification should be sought for any data, advice or recommendations contained in this book. In addition, no responsibility is assumed by the publisher for any injury and/or damage to persons or property arising from any methods, products, instructions, ideas or otherwise contained in this publication.

This publication is designed to provide accurate and authoritative information with regard to the subject matter covered herein. It is sold with the clear understanding that the Publisher is not engaged in rendering legal or any other professional services. If legal or any other expert assistance is required, the services of a competent person should be sought. FROM A DECLARATION OF PARTICIPANTS JOINTLY ADOPTED BY A COMMITTEE OF THE AMERICAN BAR ASSOCIATION AND A COMMITTEE OF PUBLISHERS.

Additional color graphics may be available in the e-book version of this book.

Library of Congress Cataloging-in-Publication Data

Child welfare : current issues, practices and challenges / editors, Alex Powell and Jenna Gray-Peterson.
       p. cm.
Includes index.
ISBN: 978-1-62257-826-9 (hardcover)
1. Child welfare. 2. Children--Services for. 3. Child health services. 4. Mental health services.
I. Powell, Alex. II. Gray-Peterson, Jenna.
HV713.C382847 2013
362.7--dc23

                                     2012031708

Published by Nova Science Publishers, Inc. † New York

CONTENTS

Preface   **vii**

Chapter 1   Mental Health Oversight for Children and Adolescents
                 in Child Welfare Custody   **1**
                 Thomas I. Mackie, Christina M. Mulé, Justeen Hyde
                 and Laurel K. Leslie

Chapter 2   Children in Foster Care and Excessive Medications   **37**
                 Jill Littrrell

Chapter 3   Protecting the Protectors: Secondary Traumatic Stress
                 in Child Welfare Professionals   **65**
                 Ginny Sprang, Carlton Craig and James J. Clark

Chapter 4   Transforming Mental Health Practice in Child-Serving Systems:
                 A statewide Model for disseminating, Implementing,
                 and Sustaining a trauma-Informed, Evidence-Based Practice   **85**
                 Patti P. van Eys, Jon S. Ebert and Richard A. Epstein

Chapter 5   Educational Vulnerability of Children and Youth
                 in Foster Care   **103**
                 Andrea Zetlin

Chapter 6   Developing a Child Welfare and Child Protection System
                 in China: UNICEF Support to the Government of China   **115**
                 Lisa Ng Bow

Chapter 7   Mindfulness Training: A Promising Approach for Addressing
                 the Needs of Child Welfare System Children and Families   **151**
                 Cynthia V. Heywood, Philip A. Fisher and Yi-Yuan Tang

Index   **181**

PREFACE

In this book, the authors present topical research in the study of the current issues, practices and challenges related to child welfare today. Topics include mental health oversight for children and adolescents in child welfare custody; children in foster care and excessive medications; youth sexuality and health conditions; secondary traumatic stress in child welfare professionals; transforming mental health practices in child-serving systems; educational vulnerability of children and youth in foster care; developing a child welfare and child protection system in China; and mindfulness training for addressing the needs of child welfare system children and families.

In this book, the authors present topical research in the study of the current issues, practices and challenges related to child welfare today. Topics include mental health oversight for children and adolescents in child welfare custody; children in foster care and excessive medications; youth sexuality and health conditions; secondary traumatic stress in child welfare professionals; transforming mental health practices in child-serving systems; educational vulnerability of children and youth in foster care; developing a child welfare and child protection system in China; and mindfulness training for addressing the needs of child welfare system children and families.

Chapter 1 – Since 1997, child welfare agencies have been increasingly held accountable by Federal and State policies to ensure the mental health needs of children in their care are met. Federal legislation, the Adoptions and Safe Families Act of 1997, extended the purview of state child welfare agencies from ensuring the safety and permanency of children to also include well-being, referring to their physical, mental, developmental, and dental health, particularly those children legally removed from the care of their parents, either temporarily or permanently (hereafter, "children in welfare custody"). Recent Federal legislation, the Fostering Connections to Success and Increasing Adoptions Act of 2008 and the Child and Family Services Innovation Act of 2011, reflect this increased commitment by mandating that state child welfare agencies develop a plan for oversight of mental health services, including mental health evaluation, appropriate psychotropic medication use, and responses to address the trauma experienced by children in child welfare custody.

This chapter will describe the level of mental health need among children involved in the child welfare/child protective services (CW/CPS) system, with a particular focus on those children removed from their home of origin and placed in child welfare custody; provide a brief legislative history of how 'well-being,' specifically mental health, fell under the purview of child welfare agencies; propose a model specifying components of and organizational resources for a mental health oversight system; and, for each component/resource, delineate the challenges confronted by state child welfare agencies, their responses, and the practice implications. The authors draw on considerable research conducted on the mental health needs and service use of children in child welfare custody, as well as interviews recently conducted with key informants from child welfare agencies in 48 States and the District of Columbia, from March 2009 until January 2010.

The chapter will conclude by discussing the organizational resources that assist child welfare agencies in ensuring mental health oversight in both policy and practice. Themes will include the importance of mental health expertise and on-going training and collaboration with other state child-serving systems (specifically, State Medicaid agencies as the primary payer of mental health services and m ental health authorities as the primary provider of mental health services). Children in child welfare custody need and deserve the best mental health services that a state can provide. Strong committed leadership from child welfare agencies, alongside stakeholder collaborations, will be critical to meeting the significant need of children in their care.

Chapter 2 – Children in foster care system are more likely to receive diagnoses of major mental illness and to be medicated with powerful medications such as antipsychotic drugs. Reasons for the increased risk of the actual mental illnesses and for the diagnoses of illness among children in foster care are reviewed. The reliabilities of various diagnoses are considered. The legitimacy of the rationale for early medications to prevent later disability is discussed. The very real hazards of medicating with antipsychotics, anticonvulsants, stimulants, mood stabilizers and antidepressants are reviewed. A discussion of advocacy efforts occurring around the United States on behalf of medicated children in the foster care system is presented. Finally, changes being instituted by the federal government through the Department of Health, Education, and Welfare and the Government Accounting Office (GAO), following the hearing of December 1, 2011 convened by Senator Thomas Carper, are discussed.

Chapter 3 – This chapter provides an overview of a study that investigates predictors of STS in a national sample of 669 professionals, highlighting and exploring the differential responses of child welfare workers. Study participants were recruited via licensure board rosters and professional membership lists in six states, and invited to participate in an online survey. All participants completed the Professional Quality of Life IV (Stamm, 2000). Findings indicate that child welfare job status, religious participation and rurality predicted higher levels of STS and Burnout in the sample. Comparisons of STS and Burnout among the other professions were nonsignificant. Strategies for improving worker self-care, and organizational approaches towards STS prevention, early intervention and treatment for child welfare agencies are provided.

Chapter 4 – Policymakers are increasingly charging public-sector child-serving systems (e.g., mental health, child welfare, juvenile justice) to implement evidence-based practices. Recent reviews reveal a relative lack of data regarding the effectiveness of specific dissemination and implementation strategies, but have identified a number of factors such as government funding and ideological support, organizational openness to change, active learning models and ongoing consultation/supervision that may be associated with effectiveness. Various conceptual models have emerged that incorporate some or all of these factors. The current chapter will begin with a review of the dissemination and implementation science literature. This review will be followed by a description of the Tennessee Trauma-

Focused Cognitive Behavioral Therapy (TF-CBT) Learning Collaborative, a statewide dissemination and implementation project led by the five Centers of Excellence for Children in State Custody in the state of Tennessee in collaboration with experts from the National Child Traumatic Stress Network and community partners. Since 2008, the Tennessee TF-CBT Learning Collaborative has trained more than 700 clinicians in 50 community mental health agencies across the state using the National Center for Child Traumatic Stress Learning Collaborative model through four 9-month learning collaborative experiences. These intensive training opportunities were followed with six booster sessions for new staff within the agencies, six advanced topic trainings for supervisors and advanced clinicians, and ongoing consultation calls for clinicians, supervisors and agency senior leaders. This presentation of the efforts in Tennessee will be followed by a discussion of the lessons learned from the Tennessee experience that may help others overcome dissemination and implementation challenges in their jurisdictions.

Chapter 5 – Bradley, an African-American 6 year old, entered the kindergarten class in March. He had just moved, mid-school year, from across the country because his birth mother lost custody of him. While his peers were practicing writing, reading and adding, Bradley struggled to write his name. When he first arrived, the school knew only that he was in foster care and had an IEP stipulating a variety of special education services. The paperwork accompanying his enrollment was sparse because his relative caregiver was given no more documentation than the school. Although multiple school employees requested records over and over again, neither Bradley's previous school nor the school district responded to these formal requests. After several months Bradley's biological mother finally sent past IEPs and several evaluation documents that provided more insight into his school history. Just as the school was getting to know Bradley, figure out his needs, and make progress toward his goals, Bradley's biological mother regained custody and he was moved back across the country (Montreuil and Zetlin,2012, p.3). Students like Bradley can be found in almost every school in the nation. Children in the foster care system, like Bradley, move from school to school and home to home with a lack of consistency. The effects of this instability can be very challenging for the foster child, caregiver, school, and child welfare agency.

Chapter 6 – China faces many complex new challenges in light of the current trends of rapid economic growth, urbanization, massive domestic migration, dislocation and separation of family members, changing family structures, increasing cost of basic social services, rising disparities, and increasing frequency of natural disasters. In this current context, children and their families are increasingly exposed to new social welfare and child protection risks, with poverty acting as a contributing factor to the risk of child protection violations. As it has become more difficult for the Chinese government to manage these risks and vulnerabilities through vertical social protection programs, China is beginning to shift from an issues-based approach to social welfare and child protection toward a more comprehensive, multisectoral child welfare and child protection system as the most effective way to address new challenges. This new system comprises a social welfare system that provides (a) universal benefits to support social protection and services for all children and their families, and within this, (b) a child protection system that targets the most vulnerable children.

UNICEF is supporting the Chinese government to strengthen its social welfare system for children at three basic levels: (a) at the upstream and national level, supporting the development of child-sensitive national social protection, social assistance and child protection policies, laws, and frameworks; (b) at the intermediate or provincial level, developing strategies, mechanisms, and plans that facilitate the implementation of national child welfare and child protection laws and policies; and (c) at the community level, piloting and demonstrating effective, affordable, and sustainable intersectoral child welfare and child protection packages and models within diverse local settings for possible government replication (this component also feeds into policy development). Within this social welfare framework, UNICEF is supporting China to move toward the establishment of a child protection system; this involves policy and legal reforms aimed at a strengthening a systems approach to child protection which is integrally linked with the social welfare and justice systems. Support is also being provided to demonstrate and develop community-based child protection service models that prevent and respond to violence, abuse, exploitation, and neglect.

Chapter 7 – Foster children often demonstrate intensive clinical needs and evidence risk for long-term difficulties as a result of adversity and maltreatment. Addressing their diverse and intensive needs can be challenging for foster caregivers and complex for their providers. Although intervention research over the past decades has yielded a number of evidence-based treatment approaches for foster children and their caregivers, enhancement and individualization continues to be needed. As the field advances, more attention is being paid to critical skills that increase competence and resilience as protective factors versus the more traditional focus on pathology. Particularly, self-regulation and attention are becoming increasingly salient foci for scientists and practitioners seeking to improve treatment effectiveness and favorable outcomes.

Mindfulness-oriented interventions pose a forum for uniquely targeting these outcomes and have the potential to (1) promote the development of self-regulation and attentional focus in foster children, (2) increase the effect of already robust therapies, (3) enhance risk prevention efforts for children whose lives are characterized by adversity, (4) address obstacles to effective and consistent implementation of therapeutic parenting strategies, and (5) increase overall well-being and quality of life for foster children and their caregivers. In this chapter, the following topics are discussed: (1) the presenting issues among foster children and their need for effective and individualized treatments, (2) the interplay of stress and neurobiology on the development critical skills, (3) current intervention trends, and (4) applications for mindfulness-oriented therapies in research and practice.

In: Child Welfare
Editors: Alex Powell and Jenna Gray-Peterson

ISBN: 978-1-62257-826-9
© 2013 Nova Science Publishers, Inc.

Chapter 1

MENTAL HEALTH OVERSIGHT FOR CHILDREN AND ADOLESCENTS IN CHILD WELFARE CUSTODY

Thomas I. Mackie[1,2], Christina M. Mulé[1,3], Justeen Hyde[4,5] and Laurel K. Leslie[1]

[1]Institute for Clinical Research and Health Policy Studies,
Tufts Medical Center, Boston, Massachusetts, US
[2]Brandeis University, Waltham, Massachusetts, US
[3]Northeastern University, Boston, Massachusetts
[4]Institute for Community Health, Cambridge, Massachusetts, US
[5]Harvard Medical School, Boston, Massachusetts, US

ABSTRACT

Since 1997, child welfare agencies have been increasingly held accountable by Federal and State policies to ensure the mental health needs of children in their care are met. Federal legislation, the Adoptions and Safe Families Act of 1997, extended the purview of state child welfare agencies from ensuring the safety and permanency of children to also include well-being, referring to their physical, mental, developmental, and dental health, particularly those children legally removed from the care of their parents, either temporarily or permanently (hereafter, "children in welfare custody"). Recent Federal legislation, the Fostering Connections to Success and Increasing Adoptions Act of 2008 and the Child and Family Services Innovation Act of 2011, reflect this increased commitment by mandating that state child welfare agencies develop a plan for oversight of mental health services, including mental health evaluation, appropriate psychotropic medication use, and responses to address the trauma experienced by children in child welfare custody.

This chapter will describe the level of mental health need among children involved in the child welfare/child protective services (CW/CPS) system, with a particular focus on those children removed from their home of origin and placed in child welfare custody; provide a brief legislative history of how 'well-being,' specifically mental health, fell under the purview of child welfare agencies; propose a model specifying components of and organizational resources for a mental health oversight system; and, for each component/resource, delineate the challenges confronted by state child welfare agencies, their responses, and the practice implications. We draw on considerable research conducted on the mental health needs and service use of children in child welfare custody, as well as interviews recently conducted with key informants from child welfare agencies in 48 States and the District of Columbia, from March 2009 until January 2010.

The chapter will conclude by discussing the organizational resources that assist child welfare agencies in ensuring mental health oversight in both policy and practice. Themes will include the importance of mental health expertise and on-going training and collaboration with other state child-serving systems (specifically, State Medicaid agencies as the primary payer of mental health services and m ental health authorities as the primary provider of mental health services).

Children in child welfare custody need and deserve the best mental health services that a state can provide. Strong committed leadership from child welfare agencies, alongside stakeholder collaborations, will be critical to meeting the significant need of children in their care.

INTRODUCTION

Children and adolescents (hereafter "children") involved with the child protective services/child welfare system (CPS/CW; see Table 1 for terms and definitions used within this chapter) represent a uniquely vulnerable and at-risk subpopulation in our nation. In 2010, the National Child Abuse and Neglect Data System (NCANDS) estimated that 695,000 children were victims of child maltreatment, of which 59,000 were repeat victims (U.S. Department of Health and Human Services [U.S. DHHS], Administration for Children and Families [ACF], Administration on Children, Youth and Families, Children's Bureau, 2011). Approximately, 78% suffered neglect, 18% were physically abused, 9% were sexually abused, 8% were psychologically maltreated, and 2% were medically neglected (U.S. DHHS, ACF, Administration on Children, Youth and Families, Children's Bureau, 2011). On any given day, approximately 423,000 children were removed from their home and placed in out-of-home care (Child Welfare Information Gateway, 2011).

Given their histories of trauma and neglect, it is not surprising that children involved with both CPS/CW are at heightened risk for mental health problems (i.e., socioemotional, behavioral, developmental, and psychiatric problems) relative to their counterparts from the general population (Burns et al., 2004; Kolko et al., 2010; Leslie et al., 2005b; Leslie, Hurlburt, Landsverk, Barth, and Slymen, 2004).

According to a recent and nationally representative study, nearly half of all involved children (i.e., children involved with CPS/CW) have clinically significant mental health problems (e.g., coping difficulties, conduct disorder, aggressive behavior, and depression being among the most common (Burns et al., 2004) compared to a rate of approximately 20% in the general population (Dore, 2005). Despite the disproportionate rates of mental health care need among involved children, research has consistently demonstrated a gap between the need and receipt of psychological services (Burns et al., 2004).

Specifically, while children with clinically significant mental health problems are more likely to receive outpatient mental health care (Burns et al., 2004; Garland, Landsverk, Hough, and Ellis-Macleod, 1996; Hurlburt et al., 2004), some studies suggest that there are also non-clinical factors that influence the use of outpatient mental health services (Burns et al., 2004; Garland et al., 2000; Garland et al., 1996; Leslie et al., 2000; Leslie et al., 2004).

Table 1. Child Welfare and Mental Health Terms and Working Definitions

Terms	Definitions
Assent	A 3-part process that includes the child understanding (to the best of his/her developmental ability) treatment options, the child voluntarily choosing to undergo treatment options, and the child communicating this choice.
Children	Children and adolescents between the ages of 0-17.
Children Involved with CPS/CW ("Involved Children")	Children involved with CPS/CW are suspected to have suffered from child abuse or neglect (CA/N). As a way to protect a child from CA/N, an investigation is conducted whereby the child/family/friends are interviewed, photographs may be taken (if necessary to document physical abuse), and home visits are conducted.
Children in Child Welfare Custody	Children who have been removed from their home out of concern for their safety and well-being. Guardianship is granted to the child welfare system and a child welfare worker works toward a permanent placement (either reunification with parent or an alternative such as kinship care or adoption) for the child.
Informed Consent	The process of the clinician providing information, including benefits and risks, to the child and designee about all possible treatments; the designee makes an informed treatment decision based on the best interest of the child. For children in child welfare custody, terminology and associated definitions also include substitute judgment and informed permission.
Mental Health Evaluation	Screening and/or assessment for emotional and behavioral problems.
Mental Health Services	Services such as evaluation, psychosocial, and psychopharmacology treatment targeting improvement of mental health outcomes.
Mental Health Problems	An emotional and/or behavioral condition generally associated with distress or a disability and not considered a part of normal development.
Psychosocial Therapy	Non-medication therapies such as cognitive, behavioral, and family systems therapies; may be used with or without psychotropic medication.
Psychotropic Medications	Broad category of medications that can alter the effect of perception, emotion, and/or behavior. In this chapter, psychotropic medications are used interchangeably with psychopharmacology.
Polypharmacy	The concomitant use of two or more medications to manage mental health problems.
Red Flags	Markers used in audits, case reviews, or databases located within child welfare, Medicaid, mental health, and managed care plans to identify cases in which available data suggest medication use may not be appropriate.
Policy/Guidelines	Policy refers to state legislation, court rules, inter- and intra-agency policy, or administrative directives. Guideline refers to written procedures that constitute formal procedure or protocol for the child welfare agency.

For example, involved children who are older, from Caucasian ancestry, and have a parent with a severe mental illness are more likely than other children involved with CP/CWS to make use of mental health services (Burns et al., 2004).

For children who are removed from their home of origin and placed into child welfare custody, high rates of mental health problems exist as well. Specifically, regional and national studies approximate that between 35% to 85% of children in child welfare custody have clinically significant or borderline mental health problems[1] (Chernoff, Combs-Orme, Risley-Curtiss, and Heisler, 1994; Clausen, Landsverk, Ganger, Chadwick, and Litrownik, 1998; Garland, Hough, Landsverk, and Brown, 2001; Halfon and Klee, 1987; Hockstadt, Jaudes, Zimo, and Schachter, 1987; Kavaler and Swire, 1983; McMillen et al., 2005; Newton, Litrownik, and Landsverk, 2000; Pilowsky, 1995; Schor, 1982). Despite high rates of mental health problems, research has consistently documented the underutilization of services (Leslie et al., 2000; Leslie et al., 2004; Romanelli et al., 2009). For example, placement type is a strong predictor of outpatient mental health service use; that is, children in non-relative placements (e.g., foster care, group, and residential settings) may be more likely to receive mental health services than those placed with relatives (e.g., kinship care; (Leslie et al., 2000; Leslie et al., 2005b; Stahmer et al., 2005). Additionally, the nature by which children enter child welfare custody is a significant predictor of mental health service use. Namely, children with a history of neglect or caregiver absence are less likely than other maltreated children (e.g., children who have been sexually victimized or physically abused) to receive services, regardless of their level of their mental health need (Garland et al., 1996; Kolko, Selelyo, and Brown, 1999). Among those placed in child welfare custody, children who entered due to a history of caregiver neglect may be less likely to receive mental health services than other maltreated children (Leslie et al., 2000). In contrast, children placed due to sexual abuse are more likely to receive services, irrespective of their level of mental health need (Garland et al., 1996).

Children in child welfare custody experience multiple transitions, including entry or re-entry into child welfare custody, changes in out-of-home placement while in custody, and aging out of the child welfare system. Up to a quarter of youth in child welfare custody receive up to three or more placement changes while in child welfare custody. About a third of youth reenter the foster care system after returning to their biological families (Schor, 1988). These transitions are marked with potential emotional trauma for the child (Littner, 1956). Therefore, transition services require particular attention, especially in facilitating mental health care services between placement transition and when transitioning out of the child welfare system.

There are numerous barriers to accessing mental health services that contribute to the underuse of care. First, because Medicaid is the primary funder of health care services for children in child welfare custody (Leslie, Kelleher, Burns, Landsverk, and Rolls, 2003b), children are limited to providers who accept Medicaid reimbursement; aidentifying these providers can be especially difficult in rural and underserved urban areas (Halfon et al., 1987; Iglehart, 2003; Yudkowsky, Cartland, and Flint, 1990). Furthermore, because children in child welfare custody experience frequent placement changes (Leslie, Kelleher, et al., 2003b), it may be difficult for them to establish a therapeutic alliance or rapport with a mental health

---

[1] The selected studies utilized different sample definitions (e.g., age ranges differed) and measurement tools (e.g., the Child Behavior Checklist [CBCL] and the Diagnostic Interview Schedule for Children [DISC-IV]).

care provider. This may hamper the possible benefits of treatment. Frequent placement changes also negatively affect care coordination for children in child welfare custody, as they necessitate increased communication among stakeholders (e.g., transfer of medical records, obtaining consent to begin psychotherapy, transportation arrangements, etc) and making new health care arrangements (e.g., re-identifying providers in the current placement location) that promote collaboration among mental health services, early intervention, schools, and primary care. Following through with these logistical matters requires time and often results in a gap in service utilization for children in child welfare custody. Finally, related to access to psychosocial treatments, the quality of the interventions provided to these children has been somewhat variable (Landsverk, Burns, Stambaugh, and Rolls-Reutz, 2006; Leslie et al., 2005a). That is, although some children are able to access treatment, interventions being carried out may not be evidence-based or empirically supported.

Since the early 1990s, concerns with potential overuse of psychotropic medications among children in child welfare custody have been associated with myriad factors, including limited coverage for inpatient and partial hospital program, limited reimbursement avenues for outpatient psychosocial services, and shortages of child and adolescent psychiatrists (Goodwin, Gould, Blanco, and Olfson, 2001; Olfson, Gameroff, Marcus, and Waslick, 2003). State Medicaid claims analyses suggest that rates of psychotropic medication use range from 37% to 52% among children in child welfare custody (Ferguson, Glesener, and Raschick, 2006; Kansas Health Policy Authority, 2009; Strayhorn, 2006), which sharply contrasts a rate of 4% in the general population (Olfson, Marcus, Weissman, and Jensen, 2002). Researchers suggest that the high rates of psychotropic medication use may be attributable to a higher prevalence of emotional and behavioral problems among children in child welfare custody (Landsverk, Garland, and Leslie, 2002); the impact of placement transitions (Battistelli, 1996); lack of transparency regarding oversight of medical and behavioral health care (i.e., mental health services (Battistelli, 1996); decline of behavioral health services (Olfson, Blanco, Liu, Moreno, and Laje, 2006); and finally, the challenges in access to and quality of Medicaid services (Iglehart, 2003). Not surprisingly, with the increased use of psychotropic medications, there are increasing concerns around specific prescribing patterns, such as polypharmacy (i.e., concomitant use of multiple medications (Zito et al., 2008) and prescriptions to children under 5 years of age (Leslie, Raghavan, Zhang, and Aarons, 2010).

Given the challenges of meeting the mental health care needs of children involved with CPS/CW regardless of their legal status, there are subsequently deleterious effects on the long-term mental health and child welfare outcomes (e.g., permanency, reunification, etc.) for these children. For example, research has demonstrated that children exiting out of the child welfare system experience mental health problems at rates much higher than those of the general population (Pecora et al., 2003). More specifically, the rates of drug dependence among alumni of the child welfare system was over seven times greater than that of the general population; post-traumatic stress disorder (PTSD) is nearly five times that of the general population; and panic disorder is over three times greater (Pecora et al., 2003). Furthermore, externalizing behavior problems (e.g., impulsivity, aggression, etc.), often linked with mental health problems, have been associated with increased placement disruptions (Newton et al., 2000), longer lengths of stay in care (Horwitz, Simms, and Farrington, 1994; Kupsinel and Dubsky, 1999), and a reduced likelihood of family reunification or adoption (Courtney and Wong, 1996; Landsverk, Davis, Ganger, Newton, and Johnson, 1996).

Legislative Response to Mental Health Care Needs

Research highlighting the challenges in meeting the mental health care needs of children in child welfare custody and the resulting negative consequences to long-term mental health outcomes has sparked a policy shift in child welfare practice. Specifically, rather than concentrating solely on the safety and permanency of children in child welfare custody, the Adoption and Safe Families Act of 1997 (P.L. 105-89) mandated for the first time that the *well-being* of children (i.e., mental, physical, developmental, and dental health; Wulczyn, Barth, Yuan, Harden, and Landsverk, 2005) be included as an element of the mission. In 2008, the Fostering Connections to Success and Increasing Adoptions Act of 2008 (P.L. 110-351) was passed as a complement to P.L. 103-382. Specifically, the new Act charges state child welfare agencies to partner with clinical practitioners and Medicaid to provide ongoing oversight of health and behavioral health services, including psychotropic medications, for children in child welfare custody.

Recent Federal legislation, Child and Family Services Improvement and Innovation Act (P.L. 112-34; 2011), took P. L. 103-382 one step further, requiring states to develop specific protocols related to the oversight of psychotropic medications for children in child welfare custody. Additionally, under the new Act, states were also required to outline in the same oversight plan how they intend to respond to emotional traumas experienced by these children (Child and Family Services Improvement and Innovation Act, 2011). Congruent with this call, Federal efforts to ensure adequate mental health oversight have largely focused on the role and responsibilities of state child welfare agencies and partnering child-serving systems in providing oversight of mental health care.

While the demonstrated commitment of the federal government is evident in recent legislation, the Government Accountability Office (GAO) has also examined mental health oversight for children in child welfare custody. In December of 2011, the GAO released a report, entitled "*HHS[2] Guidance Could Help States Improve Oversight of Psychotropic Prescriptions,*" which presented agency-derived research evidence from five states (i.e., Florida, Massachusetts, Michigan, Oregon, and Texas). The GAO report (2011) made clear that children in child welfare custody are being prescribed psychotropic drugs at much higher rates than children who are not in foster care. It also called attention to a number of concerning prescribing practices, such as prescribing five or more psychotropic medications for a single child and the prescription of psychotropic medications for children under one year of age. Monitoring programs in the five states were evaluated and fell short of meeting the best principle guidelines published by the American Academy of Child and Adolescent Psychiatry ([AACAP]; AACAP, 2011); consequently, the GAO recommended that HSS endorse guidance regarding psychotropic medication oversight for state child welfare agencies and their partners (GAO, 2011).

As a result of all of the legislative and research activity around mental health care for children in child welfare custody, a major focus of 2012 for the Administration of Children and Families (ACF) is the development and implementation of state oversight plans in response to P.L. 112-34 (2011). A series of ongoing Federal initiatives offer research evidence and technical assistance, including conference presentations, webinars, technical

---

[2] Department of Health and Human Services (HHS).

reports, and a Web-based information clearinghouse (Child Welfare Information Gateway, Children's Bureau, ACF, and U.S. DHHS, n.d.).

These initiatives have, to date, aimed to assist State child welfare agencies and partnering child-serving systems in both understanding the scope of the problem and developing the mandated plan for psychotropic medication oversight in the State Child and Family Service Plans. In addition, the Casey Family Foundation and the Annie E. Casey Foundation, two intermediary organizations with a commitment to children in child welfare custody, have supported two large meetings of relevant federal stakeholders to share research evidence and promote cross-agency collaboration in addressing this legislation; these foundations are proposing to develop a website of evidence-based practices to address mental health needs.

OVERSIGHT OF MENTAL HEALTH CARE: WHAT WE KNOW ABOUT BEST PRACTICES

Professional guidelines, peer-reviewed articles, and technical reports are available to inform the development of a systematic response to meeting the significant mental health care needs for children in child welfare custody. For this article, we reviewed guidelines issued by four professional groups, specifically psychiatry (i.e., AACAP), child welfare (i.e., the Child Welfare League of America [CWLA]), pediatrics (i.e., the American Academy of Pediatrics [AAP]), and a multi-stakeholder working group (i.e., the Child Welfare-Mental Health Best Practice Group), composed of child welfare and mental health researchers, policy makers, and parent and child advocates (AACAP, 2001; AACAP, 2011; AACAP and CWLA, 2003; AAP, Committee on Early Childhood, Adoption, and Dependent Care, 2000, 2002; AAP, District II New York State, Task Force on Health Care for Children in Foster Care, 2005; Jensen, Romanelli, Pecora, and Ortiz, 2009; Romanelli et al., 2009). Peer-reviewed articles and additional guidelines were also consulted.

To complement available guidelines and peer-reviewed articles, we also drew from our own empirical work in 2009 and 2010 that examined the oversight of mental health care for children in child welfare custody (Leslie et al., 2010). Telephone interviews were conducted with key informants in state child welfare and affiliated agencies between March 2009 and January 2010.

Respondents included medical or mental health directors, foster care administrators, and other agency staff who were knowledgeable about the oversight of mental health care, or some component of it, for children in child welfare custody. In states with inter-agency linkages, surveys were conducted with multiple key informants from the same state. The interviews inquired about current policies and guidelines in place, challenges unique to child welfare, and innovative programmatic and policy solutions. The interviewer recorded all informant responses by hand.

For analyses of interview data, quantitative methods were used to examine descriptive and numerical data related to mechanisms for mental health oversight. For qualitative data, *a priori* and emergent codes were used to identify themes. A priori codes were based on mechanisms for mental health oversight documented in a position statement from AACAP and guidance from the AAP (AACAP, 2001; AAP, 2005; AAP, 2001).

COMPONENTS OF A MENTAL HEALTH OVERSIGHT PLAN

Consistent with the call for child-focused approaches in both child welfare and mental health (AACAP and CWLA, 2003; Kaplan, Skolnik, and Turnbull, 2009), we draw on our review and research to propose a model that traces the mental health services need of children upon entering into custody of the state- or county-administered child welfare agency through transitioning out of the child welfare system (see Figure 1). Accordingly, the proposed conceptual model includes four components at the individual service level: (1) mental health evaluation (initial and periodic), (2) targeted services (psychosocial and psychopharmacology), (3) shared decision-making and consent, and (4) transition services, including youth and family involvement. Given these core components for service provision to the individual child, we also propose a population-level activity to facilitate ongoing quality improvement, specifically, monitoring evaluation, treatment, and outcomes. Finally, we include two organizational resources that assist in the delivery of child- and population-level oversight initiatives, specifically (1) mental health expertise and stakeholder training on up-to-date guidelines, and (2) multi-stakeholder collaborations.

In the remainder of this chapter we provide an overview of each component within the model presented above. We begin with a "problem statement," which provides a brief overview of some of the known challenges of a given component. We then provide an overview of guidelines for best practices, study findings, and finally, practice implications. While this chapter will identify components for oversight of mental health care services, the reader should be cautioned that these mechanisms for oversight are presented somewhat in isolation. However, in practice many of these mechanisms are mutually reinforcing and optimally occur in concert with one another.

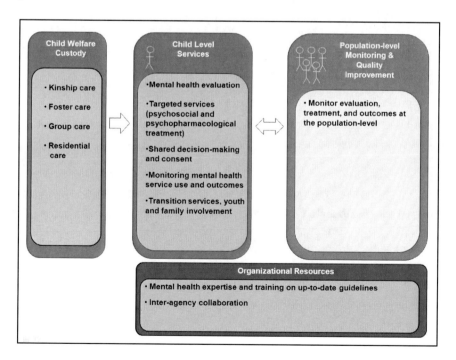

Figure 1. Oversight of Mental Health Care for Children in Child Welfare Custody.

STUDY FINDINGS: CHILD LEVEL SERVICES

Mental Health Evaluation

Problem Statement

Evaluation (i.e., screening and assessment) is a primary approach to identifying needed mental health services for children in child welfare custody (Leslie et al., 2005a). Ideally screenings and assessments are conducted with formalized or normed rating scales, semi-structured interviews with caretakers, and/or direct observations; however, research has suggested that screenings and assessments may rely more heavily on clinical judgment (Leslie et al., 2005a).

Evaluations (both screening and assessments) for mental health problems have not consistently and uniformly been conducted for children involved with CPS/CW (Leslie et al., 2005a; Leslie et al., 2003a). Research in the early 2000's found that although 94% of child welfare agencies had policies regarding the physical assessment of all children entering CPS/CW, only half of those agencies had formal policies for mental health assessments (Leslie et al., 2005a).

In addition to the lack of formalized policies around mental health evaluation, there is concern that individuals responsible for conducting screenings and assessments (i.e., child welfare staff, primary care providers) may lack the sufficient mental health training to identify children with mental health needs and, subsequently, make appropriate referrals to mental health care professionals (e.g., psychologists, psychiatrists, etc.; Burns et al., 2004; Leslie et al., 2005a; Leslie et al., 2003a). Finally, mental health clinicians conducting evaluations may also lack sufficient training in the unique circumstances and clinical needs of children in child welfare custody, potentially misevaluating the antecedents for certain behaviors.

Guidelines

Professional guidelines, peer-reviewed articles, and current child welfare policy and practice address the need for mental health evaluation, including initial and periodic evaluations for children in child welfare custody (AACAP and CWLA, 2003; AAP, District II New York State, Task Force on Health Care for Children in Foster Care, 2005; Jensen et al., 2009).

Guidelines emphasize the routine use of mental health evaluations upon entry into child welfare custody, including an initial mental health screen within 24 to 72 hours and comprehensive mental health assessment within 30-60 days of entry (AACAP and CWLA, 2003; AAP, District II New York State, Task Force on Health Care for Children in Foster Care, 2005; Jensen et al., 2009).

It should be noted that while the use of an initial mental health screen and comprehensive mental health assessment is endorsed by the three guidelines reviewed, variation exists across the guidelines with regard to specificity on the characteristics of the evaluation tools recommended, the timeframe for administration of the tool, and the recommended administrators of these evaluations (see Table 2). Each of the guidelines emphasize the need to document the identified needs and to communicate these across the multiple stakeholders involved in the care of a child.

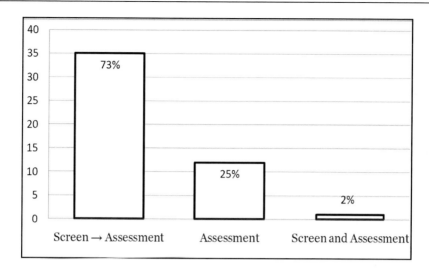

Figure 2. Mental Health Evaluation for Children in Child Welfare Custody (2009-2010).

Two guidelines specifically reference the ability for states to use Medicaid's Early Periodic Screening Diagnosis and Treatment (EPSDT) funding as a mechanism for acquiring health screenings; the EPSDT mandate in Section 1905 specifically requires regular screen for physical and behavioral health conditions, including mental and development health of the child, as well as substance use (AACAP, 2001; AAP, District II New York State, Task Force on Health Care for Children in Foster Care, 2005). Finally, the guidelines examined did not specify any recommendations regarding the population-level monitoring systems necessary to ensure receipt of the initial mental health screen and evaluation at-entry.

Study Findings

In our study, evaluation was identified as a major priority area. Respondents commented on the importance of developing mechanisms to screen and/or assess all children for mental health problems, as stated in the guidelines developed by AACAP, AAP, and the CWLA (see Table 2). For example, one child welfare administrator from the national study noted, "All of our initiatives [must] make sure that…[treatments]… flow from accurate screening and assessments." However, in 2009-2010, state child welfare agencies varied in components of the mental health evaluation systems employed. The majority of states employed a mental health screen for all children entering child welfare custody, and a mental health assessment only if indicated by a positive screen (see Figure 2). A quarter of the states employed a mental health assessment without an initial health screen, while one state employed both the screen and assessment for all children at-entry. Notably, no key informants reported that their respective state employed a two-stage screening process for all children entering child welfare custody as recommended by the multi-stakeholder working group in the Mental Health Guidelines for Child Welfare Practice (Jensen et al., 2009)

Screening and assessment tools (e.g., rating scales, semi-structured interviews, etc.) varied across states. However, some states required that specific assessment instruments be used, whereas other states gave the evaluators the liberty to choose their own assessment tools (i.e., evaluators could tailor their battery of assessment tools to the presenting referral concern).

Table 2. Mental Health Evaluation Guidelines

Mental Health Evaluation	AAP	AACAP/CWLA	Mental Health Guidelines: CW Practice
Mental Health Screen			
The screen should be…	• Standardized across the CW[4] system	• Developmentally and culturally appropriate • Sensitive to experiences of CW placement	• Sensitive to experiences of child welfare placement; and • Include stage 2 evidence-based screen.
After entry, the screen should be completed within…	• 24 hours	• 24 hours	• 72 hours for initial screen; and • 30 days for Stage 2 screen
The screen should be administered by…	• CW staff or primary care provider	• Qualified professionals with access to mental health consultation	• Caseworkers; and • Mental health professional for Stage 2 screen.
Mental Health Assessment			
The assessment should be…	• Standardized across the CW system	• Developmentally and culturally appropriate	• Evidence based
After entry, the assessment should be completed within…	• 30 days	• 60 days	• 60 days
The assessment should be administered by…	• Qualified health care professional	• Mental health provider, and • Child and adolescent psychiatrist	• Qualified mental health provider
The assessment should be conducted for…	• Children with a positive mental health screen	• Children with a positive mental health screen	• Children with a positive mental health screen

Note. AAP = American Academy of Pediatrics; AACAP = American Academy of Child and Adolescent Psychiatry; CWLA = Child Welfare League of America; CW = child welfare.

States also varied on the necessary background and training of evaluators. Across states, administrators of the evaluations came from wide-ranging disciplines (e.g., child welfare workers, mental health counselors, pediatricians, family doctors, early intervention specialists, or psychologists), which likely resulted in varying degrees of evaluation training and experience attending to the unique needs of children in child welfare custody. As expected, states' opinions varied regarding the degree of mental health expertise necessary to conduct valid screens and assessments.

The majority of state child welfare agencies ($n = 30$, 70%) reported monitoring the receipt of the mental health evaluation, with particular attention to the provision of these evaluations within the state-specific timeframes. States employed a variety of different mechanisms for tracking this information, including information management systems (child welfare, mental health), claims data (Medicaid) and in qualitative case reports. Respondents suggested variation in the extent to which this information was routinely collected and/or reviewed to identify gaps in the provision of mental health evaluations.

Practice Implications

States implemented several practices to help ensure for timely and valid evaluations, including:

- *Adoption of recommendations* put forth in AACAP, AAP, and CWLA guidelines in agency-wide protocols and procedures.
- *Screening* for emergent risk of mental health issues with 72 hours of entry into child welfare.
- *Conducting a more thorough screening* (with subsequent evaluations for those children with positive screens) or *completing a comprehensive mental health assessment* within 30-60 days following entry into foster care.
- Recommending the use of a *standardized evaluation tool.*
- Performing *routine screenings and assessments* at least once per year, as well as when significant behavioral, environmental, or other *major changes occurr* (e.g., placement change, court hearing, behavior change, transition out of care).

Targeted Services: Psychosocial and Psychopharmacologic Treatments

Problem Statement

As reviewed earlier in this chapter, multiple barriers exist in ensuring that the full range of both psychosocial and psychotropic treatments considered and used for children in child welfare custody. As described above, concerns exist around the appropriate use of psychosocial and psychotropic medication treatments, including both under- and over-use.

Guidelines

Professional organizations recommend considerations of the mental health, developmental, and educational needs when making treatment plans for youth in child welfare custody (AACAP, 2001; AACAP and CWLA, 2003; AAP, District II New York State, Task Force on Health Care for Children in Foster Care, 2005). The AAP presents the need for services across these sectors as they are "inextricably linked." All of the relevant guidelines reviewed highlighted the importance of ensuring services that address the immediate and ongoing effects of disruption and attachment, and reactions to the unfamiliar settings (AACAP, 2001; AAP District II and Task Force on Health Care for Children in Foster Care, 2005; Jensen et al., 2009; Romanelli et al., 2009). In this chapter, we draw particular attention to the mental health services while recognizing the importance of multiple modalities and interdisciplinary approaches to meeting the mental health needs of children in child welfare custody. (See *Fostering Health: Health Care for Children and Adolescents in Foster Care, 2ⁿᵈ Ed* for recommendations specific to developmental and educational services (AAP, District II New York State, Task Force on Health Care for Children in Foster Care, 2005).

Child welfare agencies are urged by available guidelines to ensure individualized, strength-based, and evidence-based treatments (EBTs) are available to clients when clinically indicated (AACAP, 2001; AACAP, 2009; Romanelli et al., 2009). In the absence of EBTs for certain pediatric mental health conditions, the Child Welfare and Mental Health Best Practices Working Group emphasizes the use of promising interventions, and adherence by mental health providers to an evidence-based practice approach (Romanelli et al., 2009). Recommendations also cite that treatment occur under the supervision of a Board eligible/certified child and adolescent psychiatrist. Such psychiatrists should have the necessary medical-based education and training, as well as the experiences necessary to consider both biological and psychosocial needs of children in child welfare custody (AACAP, 2001).

Particular attention has been given to the use of psychopharmacology (i.e., psychotropic medications) among children in child welfare custody (AACAP, 2011). Guidelines specific to psychopharmacology highlight the role of psychotropic medications as part of comprehensive mental health plan, including appropriate evaluation and psychosocial services, and longitudinal treatment planning. The guidelines recommend mental health providers, in collaboration with stakeholders, employ effective medication management systems (i.e., identification of target systems at baseline, monitoring response to treatment, and screening for side effects (AACAP, 2001). While one guideline emphasizes the role of the mental health provider in ensuring ongoing medication management AACAP, 2001), another highlights the role of the child welfare system in ensuring ongoing documentation of the child's response, side effects, risks and benefits, and timeframe for expected responses (Romanelli et al., 2009). Taken together, collaborative efforts are critical to ensure coordinated, integrated, and ongoing source of health care (frequently referred to as the "medical home") is in place.

Study Findings

Respondents from our study emphasized the need for information regarding psychosocial therapies for children in child welfare (see Figure 4). In particular, respondents felt that behavioral issues for children in child welfare custody might reflect a number of situational factors (e.g., past history of trauma, placement change, poor fit between child and caregiver) that needed to be addressed. Respondents reported that these situational factors led to challenges in ensuring that treatment provided to children matched the individual child's mental health needs.

Additionally, although some respondents recognized the benefit of medication use for some mental health problems, they wanted access to up-to-date guidelines about psychotropic medication use among children in child welfare custody. One child welfare administrator noted "[We] need guidelines to determine whether medications are needed, and if so, for how long." Respondents felt that this information was needed across stakeholder groups including children, caregivers, child welfare workers and administrators, prescribers, and other child-serving organizations (e.g., schools, residential facilities;see later section on Organizational Resources: Mental health expertise and training on up-to-date guidelines).

Practice Implications

States employed several approaches for improving access to quality psychosocial and psychopharmacological treatments, as well as strengthening the mechanisms of which they use for oversight. Their approaches included:

- Finding *reliable, up-to-date sources of information about clinical care*, both for psychosocial and psychopharmacologic treatments.
- *Partnering with professional organizations* to provide clear guidance to prescribers about standards of care using AACAP guidelines, practice parameters, and other resources.
- *Partnering with Medicaid*, mental health agencies, or academic centers to provide feedback to "outliers."
- Hiring staff or or working with co-located Medicaid or mental health *staff with mental health expertise* within the child welfare system.
- Developing *tele-psychotherapy and –psychiatry* programs to address shortages of specialists in rural areas.
- *Consulting with pediatric and mental health experts* interested in children in child welfare custody who work outside the child welfare system. Experts included clinicians at a local community public health department or mental health agency, or researchers at an academic medical center with interests in children in child welfare custody (see Organizational Resources: Mental health expertise and training on up-to-date guidelines).
- *Developing a referral network* of primary care and mental health clinicians with expertise in child welfare.
- *Establishing placement specialists* in child welfare to work with foster parents around behaviors that result in placement changes.

Shared Decision-Making and Consent

Problem Statement

When parental care and protection are unavailable, the child welfare agency, acting as *in loco parentis* or "in place of the parent," assumes legal responsibilities and functions of the parent. Local government agencies are bound by law to ensure that children in child welfare custody receive the services necessary to optimize their mental health (AAP, District II New York State, Task Force on Health Care for Children in Foster Care, 2005). This includes ensuring a meaningful process by which the child welfare agency or a designee of it consents to the use of mental health services, both psychosocial and pharmacological treatments, for children in custody. Given the increased rates of mental health service use among children in child welfare custody and resource constraints of child welfare agencies, these agencies are frequently challenged by determining a meaningful and efficient informed consent approach (Naylor et al., 2007).

Guidelines

Guidelines emphasize that child welfare agencies require systems to ensure for shared decision-making between the youth, the family (biological parents, foster parent, or caregivers), and the state-assigned decision-maker (caseworker, court personnel, etc.) about treatment options, whether they be psychosocial or psychopharmacology.

Figure 3 illustrates the process by which stakeholders inform the decision-maker, who in turn may be required to have the decision authorized by a third party. Once made and authorized, appropriate stakeholders are notified of the decision. The AACAP position statement specifically recommends training requirements for child welfare, court personnel, and/or foster parents to help them become more effective advocates when informing or making treatment decisions (AACAP, 2011).

Guidelines also emphasize that mental health expertise and training be offered to the decision-maker and authorizing agent for mental health treatment (AACAP, 2011; Romanelli et al., 2009). For psychotropic medications in particular, an AACAP position statement emphasizes the need for the authorizing individual/institution to have access to a second opinion from an individual with mental health expertise (AACAP, 2011).

Study Findings

As illustrated in Figure 4, decision-making authority in states between 2009 and 2010 varied. This authority resided in several states at the clinical encounter with the prescriber, caregiver, and child participating in the process. The majority of states employed child welfare workers, supervisors or administrators, or internal units with mental health expertise with this authority.

Given concern around administration of psychotropic medications, two states relied on the Court system to approve the use of some (i.e., antipsychotics) or all psychotropic medications (Naylor et al., 2007).

Some child welfare agencies delegated authority to a specific stakeholder group depending on characteristics of the review, such as type of mental health service use (e.g., psychotropic medication use, 'extraordinary treatment,' etc.), the placement type of youth in custody (e.g., youth in residential care, youth in kinship care), or the age of the youth (e.g., 14 years or older, 18 years or older, etc.)

States relying on expert units internal or external to child welfare, or who used the Court system, prioritized more systematic approaches for obtaining informed consent. Standardized procedures were employed by some of these states for the documentation of mental health need and treatment approach, secondary review, and notification of results. Many states recognized the need for the decision-maker providing informed consent to have access to consultation to mental health expertise (see Figure 4). For example, the Guardianship Administrator of the state child welfare agency in Illinois designates an "Authorized Agent" as the individual *authorized* to consent for the use of psychotropic medications among children in child welfare custody.

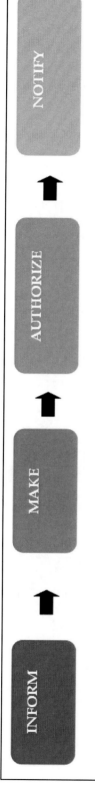

INFORM

A decision-maker is *informed* about the mental health history (when available) of the youth, the presenting emotional or behavioral problem(s), and the treatment plan. Multiple stakeholders should inform approach taken by decision-maker.

MAKE

The decision-maker (or another party) then *makes* the decision to provide informed consent for mental health treatment. At specific ages, it may be required for youth to consent, in addition to or in replacement of the typically designated decision-maker. The decision- maker may receive *consultation* from a mental health expert.

AUTHORIZE

A third party may *authorize* particular mental health treatments, such as psychotropic medications. The third party may be the court system, an expert panel internal to child welfare, or a state agency such as Medicaid. The authority may also receive *consultation* from a mental health expert.

NOTIFY

Relevant stakeholders are *notified* of the decision to begin psychotropic medications. Notification can include: name of the medication(s); **targeted** symptoms; risks, benefits, and side effects.

Figure 3. Shared Decision-making and Consent.

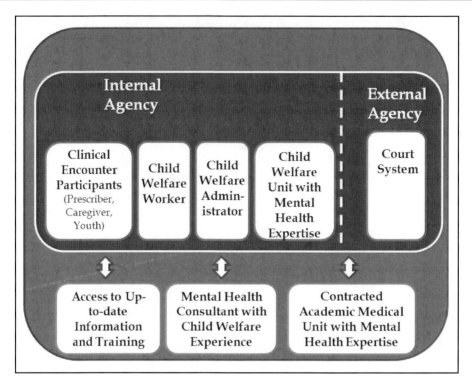

Figure 4. Informed Consent and Consultation.

According to policy, the Agent will receive a recommendation from a contracted academic medical center within 24-48 hours of a request for authorization; in this capacity, the medical center serves as a *consultant* to the agency (Child Welfare Information Gateway, Children's Bureau, ACF, and U.S. DHHS, n.d.). Whichever approach was utilized required balancing the advantages of a centralized and systematic consent process and the ability to personalize a child's mental health care.

Practice Implications
States child welfare agencies employed a variety of solutions to ensure shared decision-making and informed consent, including:

- Developing standardized protocols for informed decision-making/consent, including assent and/or consent of older youth (see Figure 4).
- Generating the capacity for a consultation in complex cases (i.e., cases that repeatedly trigger "red flags," or cases in which the child is not responding to standard treatment approaches).
- Facilitating ongoing communication (through Child and Family Team Meetings and other venues) among children, caregivers, other stakeholders who understand the child's behavioral/emotional needs best, and the people who are authorized decision-makers to assure that the treatment plan is appropriate and well implemented.
- Mandatory monitoring and periodic reporting of benefits and side effects of mental health treatments with relevant stakeholders for theindividual child in child welfare custody.

Child-Level Monitoring

Problem Statement.

A considerable literature documents the large gap between what is known in research studies about effectiveness of psychosocial and psychopharmacological interventions and what is found in the mental health service settings where children in child welfare custody receive their care (e.g., Aarons and Palinkas, 2007; Raghavan, Bright, and Shadoin, 2008). Moreover, numerous challenges, as described earlier, exist in providing mental health treatments to youth in child welfare custody, including limited access to mental health providers, multiple placement changes, and a limited evidence base to inform mental health treatment decisions for children with complex traumatic experiences, especially in psychopharmacology (Halfon et al., 1987; Leslie et al., 2003b; Yudkowsky et al., 1990). In addition to the inherent responsibility given the role of the agency as *in loco parentis,* these specific challenges in mental health care for youth in child welfare custody underscore the need for child welfare agencies to assess both service utilization and outcomes for each child in custody of the child welfare agency.

Guidelines

Guidelines emphasize the importance of monitoring various aspects of (1) service utilization, especially periodic reviews of psychotropic medication use, and (2) outcomes, including those related to mental health and functioning, placement stability, permanency, and client satisfaction (AACAP, 2011; Romanelli et al., 2009). These data may arrive from a variety of sources such as individual case reviews, audits, databases, or a combination of these sources. Guidelines recommend data acquisition from a variety of youth-serving sectors, including child welfare, Medicaid, managed care entities, and mental health departments, as well as the need for systematic review of available data.

Study Findings

In our 2009-2010 study, we identified available data sources and systematic strategies to monitor psychotropic medication use. Notably, more than a third of the states acquired, or had the potential to acquire, data from multiple databases to facilitate monitoring, whether at the child- or population-level, while about one quarter used no databases to review psychotropic medications (see Figure 5). Most states struggled with uniform data entry into their child welfare information system (e.g., State Automated Child Welfare Information System) because of the time and responsibility demands of frontline workers. Some had staff dedicated to coordinating mental health care who entered these data. Many states were interested in sharing data across public agencies.

A major challenge was the lack of "cross-talk" between different public data sources (e.g., SACWIS, Medicaid, mental health, managed care). Some states were able to access data in real time to inform specific cases; others could only access a summary of data collected over a previous time period. As described in Figure 6, available data monitoring approaches may inform client-level services prospectively (i.e., before a medication was prescribed) or retrospectively (i.e., after a medication was prescribed). Prospective mental health service reviews include optional consultation for mental health providers by child and adolescent psychiatrists ideally with child welfare experience, mandatory second opinions from a mental health provider (Naylor et al., 2007), or prior authorization based on the medication regimen requested (e.g., polypharmacy, or psychotropic medication for a child under age of 5).

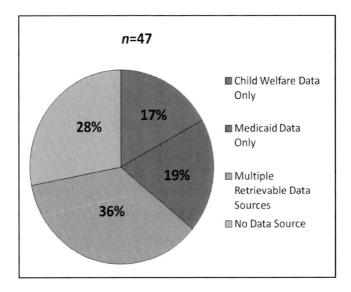

Figure 5. Databases available to state child welfare agencies.

Prospective	Retrospective
Voluntary Consultation	Court Hearings
Mandatory Second Opinion	Team Meetings
Prior Authorization	Drug Utilization Review

Figure 6. Examples of Data Monitoring Approaches.

Retrospective monitoring systems were employed to review mental health service use after administration. Examples included periodic court hearings to assess the mental health and appropriate service use for an individual child or drug utilization reviews for the individual child, frequently conducted through Medicaid claims. In both cases, these reviews could occur routinely, periodically with routine timelines for review, or on an *ad hoc* basis. The retrospective approaches also could involve analyses of data trends to inform trends occurring across populations of children in child welfare custody (e.g., placement types, geographic areas, ages, gender, race/ethnicity, etc.).

In both prospective and retrospective reviews, child welfare agencies employed red flags to monitor prescription safety and quality. Of the 48 states that participated in the national study, just over half (53%) of states used at least one "red flag" marker delineated in our interview guide (see Table 3). These markers were used in audits, case reviews, or data print-outs from databases located within child welfare, Medicaid, mental health, and managed care plans. In addition to the "red flag" markers that were asked about in the interview, just over a tenth (12.8%) used other "red flags." These included the use of any *pro re nata* (PRN) medications (i.e., the use of medications is not scheduled but administration is provided on "as needed" basis by mental health provider/caregiver) or the use of PRN medications two or more times in one week, and side effects such as weight gain or loss.

Table 3. "Red Flag" Markers

"Red Flag"	# (%) of states that endorsed
Use of psychotropic medications in young children (states varied in cutoff from 3-6 years of age)	22 (46.8%)
Polypharmacy before monopharmacy (i.e., the use of multiple medications before the use of a single medication)	10 (21.3%)
Use of multiple psychotropic medications simultaneously (states varied in cutoff from 3-5 medications)	18 (38.3%)
Use of multiple medications within the same class for longer than 30 days, including: 2-3 or more antidepressants; 2 or more antipsychotics; 2 or more stimulants (not including long-acting and short-acting stimulants); or 3 or more mood stabilizers	18 (38.3%)
Dosage exceeds current maximum recommendations (e.g., manufacturer, professional, federal, or internal state guidelines developed by state-convened panels)	14 (29.8%)
Medications not consistent with current recommendations (e.g., professional or internal state guidelines developed by state-convened panels)	14 (29.8%)
Use of newer, non-approved medications over FDA-approved medications	8 (17.0%)
Primary care doctor prescribing for a disorder other than Attention Deficit Hyperactivity Disorder, Oppositional Defiant Disorder, Adjustment Reaction, or Depression	8 (17.0%)
Antipsychotic medication use for longer than 2 years (if not diagnosed with Bipolar Disorder, Psychosis, or Schizophrenia)	8 (17.0%)
No documentation of discussion of risks and benefits of medication	10 (21.3%)

At the child-level, these "red flags" served multiple purposes, including: prompting case reviews, ordering lab work when indicated for specific medications, or initiating the prior authorization process from Medicaid for select medications.

Practice Implications

State child welfare agencies employed specific strategies to assist in monitoring child-level outcomes, including the development of:

- *A centralized system* within child welfare for informed consent. This helped eliminate delays, provided a prospective review process, and provided a database through which to track youth receiving mental health treatments, especially psychotropic medications.
- *A tracking system* using the best available data (e.g., SACWIS, Medicaid, mental health, managed care, audits) in order to get *accurate, timely retrospective data* on prescribing patterns of concern (e.g., red flags, or outliers) in mental health treatment for individual children in child welfare custody.

Transition Services, and Family and Youth Involvement

Problem Statement

As mentioned previously, transitions can be difficult for children while in child welfare custody. In addition, transitions out of care for these youthare critical to address. Prior research suggests that youth, ages 14-21 either in child welfare custody or receiving services, are not adequately engaged in mental health service delivery. Research in three Midwestern States and Missouri found that youth in child welfare custody perceive they have little voice in their own care as decisions about treatments are made by a number of adults in their lives, including foster parents, social workers, mental health professionals, and judges (Courtney and Dworsky, 2006; Courtney, Piliavin, Grogan-Kaylor, and Nesmith, 2001; McMillen et al., 2005; McMillen and Tucker, 1999). Most of these youth have limited mental health literacy and do not understand their diagnoses, available treatments (both psychosocial and pscyhopharmacology), or the risks and benefits of the mental health treatment received. In addition, continued access to intensive mental health services, including psychotropic medications, has been identified as a major problem for youth formerly in child welfare custody (Davies and Wright, 2008).

Limited mental health literacy is a particular challenge for children in child welfare custody. Mental health literacy is defined as "knowledge and beliefs about mental disorders which aid a person's recognition, management or prevention" (Jorm, 2000). Mental health literacy consists of several components, including: a) the ability to recognize specific disorders or different types of psychological distress, b) knowledge and beliefs about risk factors and causes, c) knowledge and beliefs about treatment options, d) beliefs about professional help, e) knowledge of how to seek mental health information, f) and skills to advocate for oneself within clinical settings (Jorm, 2000). Since mental health disorders are pervasive among children in child welfare custody, mental health literacy is an essential life skill (Rickwood, Deane, Wilson, and Ciarrochi, 2005). The poor developmental trajectory for this population underscores the necessity of improving mental health literacy and on-going, supported access to mental health services as these children transition to adulthood. In response, guidelines specify the importance of youth involvement to inform the mental health treatment decisions while in child welfare custody.

Similar concerns have been raised about the needs of both temporary and permanent caregivers. Foster parents often act as the primary intervention agent, given their close proximity to the child living in their home. Several evidence-based innovative, mental health treatments actually target foster parents to develop their ability to treat the child's mental health needs by providing a safe, secure, and therapeutic environment (e.g., Horwitz, Chamberlain, Landsverk, and Mullican, 2010).

Similarly, biological parents also need assistance to be involved and informed about their child's care. In 2010, 51% of children existing child welfare custody were reunified with biological parents or the primary caretaker (U.S. DHHS, ACF, Administration on Children, Youth and Families, Children's Bureau, 2011). The knowledge of the biological parent about the child, the family circumstances and cultural context offers important information for both the mental health evaluation and appropriate treatment planning (Romanelli et al., 2009). Moreover, prior research indicates that children' emotional and behavioral problems frequently escalate after returning to the biological family. Therefore, attention to educating the parents about the developmental and mental health needs of their child and appropriate therapeutic strategies for use at reunification may assist in anticipating and preventing additional morbidity (Landsverk et al., 1996).

Guidelines

Guidelines emphasize multiple components to facilitate transition services as well as youth and family involvement at the child- and case-levels, including information coordination, youth involvement and family involvement.

First, the role of medical information systems to facilitate coordination of care across placement transitions is emphasized in the reviewed guidelines (AACAP and CWLA, 2003; AAP et al., 2002). Guidelines issued by the AAP specifically reference the use of an abbreviated health record, referred to as a "medical passport" (Simms and Kelly, 1991). The form is retained by the child's caregiver to facilitate coordination of care between physical and mental health providers. In addition to these hard copy forms, child welfare agencies are increasingly building upon available child welfare, Medicaid, and mental health information systems to facilitate incorporation of electronically available data into practice (see section on Child-level Monitoring for additional details). Moreover, access to a single record of medical information that can travel between placements or is held in a single location (i.e., coordinated medical practice) despite where the child may be residing has been recommended to promote positive outcomes for children in child welfare custody (Leslie et al., 2003b). Particular attention should be made to ensure the same level of privacy and confidentiality of electronic health information systems are maintained as those in place for the written documentation.

Second, guidelines recommend state child welfare agencies make proactive efforts to involve youth, including discussions about the diagnosis, risks and benefits, and potential adverse effects of the medications (AACAP, 2011; Romanelli et al., 2009). The Child Welfare and Mental Health Best Practices Group emphasizes that the prescriber serve as a consultant to the child, parents, caretakers, and child welfare staff (Romanelli et al., 2009). Ultimately, the child and caregiver will be responsible for implementing treatment so their involvement is critical.

Third, guidelines emphasize the involvement of biological families, when possible. Prior research suggests that benefits exist when parents who have maltreated their children participate in mental health care for their children, including lower rates of re-abuse (Chaffin and Friedrich, 2004). Both information coordination and training are important to assist in maintaining the involvement of biological parents. Information coordination includes the provision of the "medical passport" or something equivalent, as described earlier, to facilitate communication while in child welfare custody, when appropriate, and in reunification, if achieved.

Study Findings

Our national study suggests that child welfare agencies have policies and practices in place that demonstrate a commitment to youth and family involvement. As one child welfare administrator stated, "[We need] to involve families and youth, when age-appropriate, in decisions about the child...we also need better training for youth about diagnoses and medications." A number of states were pioneering the development of youth mental health guides co-created with children in child welfare custody. Despite these efforts (as described in practice implications below), challenges to ensuring ongoing youth and family involvement were also noted. Agencies were challenged to provide adequate training and education to children about mental health treatments. This was of particular concern for youth transitioning out of the foster care system. Concerns were also expressed about the lack of involvement of birth parents and/or guardians in the informed consent process. Many expressed interest in implementing a family-centered approach, in part to help increase the involvement of birth parents and other key stakeholders. Involvement of biological parents from the beginning was seen as particularly important if family reunification is a goal. A child welfare administrator from our national study noted, "Keep families involved because they need to be willing to keep the care going after reunification. [We] need to keep in mind the long-run when dealing with these issues − not only where the child came from but also where he/she is going."

Practice Implications

States employed multiple solutions to ease transitions and to facilitate youth and family involvement, including:

- *Educating* all stakeholders about medications and about psychiatric diagnoses and treatment options.
- Providing *ongoing information to children, youth, and families* about diagnoses, effective treatment options, and managing care throughout life.
- Developing a *transition plan* for youth aging out of foster care that specifically addressed *engaging the youth* in managing their own symptoms and treatments and *identifying who will prescribe medications* once out of care.
- Developing a youth handbook for youth in child welfare custody. Some of these are co-authored by other alumni of the child welfare system, alongside mental health and child welfare experts; youth are able to draw from their own experiences in ensuring an accessible and relevant resource. For examples, see National Resource Center for Permanency and Family Connections (NRCPFC, 2012).
- *Hosting "brown bag" call-in sessions*, led by medical or mental health experts in child welfare, for foster parents, biological parents, and youth about mental health issues and treatments, including medications.

STUDY FINDINGS: POPULATION LEVEL SERVICES

Monitor Mental Health Evaluation, Treatment, and Outcomes at the Population-Level

Problem Statement

Contact with child welfare is a gateway into outpatient mental health services for children in child welfare custody (Leslie et al., 2005b). Despite relatively high rates of service utilization, concerns remain with regard to the appropriate receipt of mental health evaluations and treatments, specifically *access* to and *quality* of available services. As reviewed earlier, prior research suggests children in child welfare custody may not receive access to mental health evaluations consistent with policies or guidelines (Leslie et al., 2005a).

Moreover, concerns around the quality of psychosocial and pharmacological treatments have been expressed (dosReis, Zito, Safer, and Soeken, 2001; Zito et al., 2008). In a national probability sample of child welfare service areas, Leslie and colleagues (Leslie et al., 2011) demonstrated rates of medication use from zero to 40% between child protective service agency service areas, a 40-fold variation among children involved with CW/CPS. Moreover, of 472 youth in foster care prescribed at least one psychotropic medication in one state, 41% received three or more psychotropic medications concomitantly (Zito et al., 2008).

Guidelines

Given concerns of access and quality of mental health services, guidelines emphasize the importance of monitoring trends in both service use and outcomes retrospectively at the population-level. Monitoring of service use allows child welfare agencies to specify practice patterns of concern and to identify any outliers or red flags (see Table 1 for terms and definitions) (AACAP, 2011; Romanelli et al., 2009). Patterns of psychotropic medication use could be evaluated at the aggregate population level or on a prescriber-specific basis, with necessary action taken in response to prescribing patterns of concern. In addition to monitoring service use, guidelines specify the importance of tracking outcomes, at the aggregate level, including psychosocial functioning and client satisfaction, two measures typical of mental health care, and placement stability and permanency, both critical to the child welfare mission (Romanelli et al., 2009).

Study Findings

Respondents indicated that population-level monitoring facilitated an improved understanding of the extent and scope of a problem related to mental health services (e.g., psychotropic medication use) among children in child welfare custody. States used autonomous and/or linked databases available from child welfare (e.g., SACWIS), Medicaid, mental health agencies, and managed care plans (see Figure 7). Respondents indicated challenges in accessing population-level data from their own databases as well as those of other youth-serving agencies (such as Medicaid, mental health, and the Judiciary). For example, respondents suggested there was a lack of recognition concerning rates of psychotropic medication use due to limited data at the local- and state- level about psychotropic medication use among children in child welfare custody. Respondents indicated particular challenges in acquiring quality and timely data to track medication use at the population level. When population-level monitoring systems were accessible for periodic review and data were reliable, the population-level monitoring systems were frequently used to conduct analyses at the child-, prescriber-, and population -levels.

Practice Implications

States employed multiple solutions to ease transitions and to facilitate population-level monitoring, including:

- *Developing a tracking system* using the best available data (e.g., SACWIS, Medicaid, mental health, managed care, audits) in order to get *accurate, timely data* on prescribing trends for youth in the child welfare system.

- *Contracting* with academic medical centers or other entities *to collect and analyze aggregate data* on a periodic basis, using state or grant funding.
- *Working with other systems* to find staff to track medication use (e.g., public health nurses, Medicaid pharmacy staff).

STUDY FINDINGS: ORGANIZATIONAL RESOURCES

Mental Health Expertise and Training on Up-to-Date Guidelines

Problem Statement

Because historically child welfare agencies have focused on "safety" and "permanency," child welfare agencies may struggle to garner access to the expertise in mental health necessary to fulfill recent mandates for mental health oversight (Wulczyn et al., 2005). Moreover, the requirements for additional mental health oversight have been accompanied with few financial resources to assist in building human resource capital, whether acquiring mental health expertise or providing training on mental health needs and services, to inform mental health care planning and implementation. As a result, child welfare agencies are challenged to ensure (1) adequate mental health expertise at the child- and population-level to inform policy and practice development, implementation, and quality improvement and (2) training on up-to-date guidelines for the myriad stakeholders involved in the care of children in child welfare custody.

Guidelines

The creation of the guidelines from professional groups, such as AAP and AACAP, are testament to the importance and value placed on having mental health expertise inform policy development and implementation in mental health oversight systems at the child- and population-level (AACAP, 2009; AAP, District II New York State, Task Force on Health Care for Children in Foster Care, 2005). In the guidelines, specific attention is provided to ensuring appropriately qualified mental health providers assist at both levels. The guidelines emphasize the importance of qualified mental health expertise for aspects of policy development and service delivery, including mental health evaluation and mental health services, with particular focus on psychotropic medication oversight. The guidelines provide criteria for those mental health professionals qualified to administer mental health evaluations (see Table 2 for additional details). Additionally, the AACAP position statement posits that a child and adolescent psychiatrist administer a program to oversee the utilization of medications for youth in child welfare custody (AACAP, 2011).

Study Findings

As depicted in Figure 6, almost two-thirds (60%) of state child welfare agencies interviewed had a medical director or mental health director; more specifically, almost a tenth (8%) a medical director alone, just over a quarter a mental health director alone (26%), and just over a quarter (26%) with both. In analyses, staffing both a medical and mental health director was associated with presence of policies/guidelines for the oversight of psychotropic medications (Mackie et al., 2011).

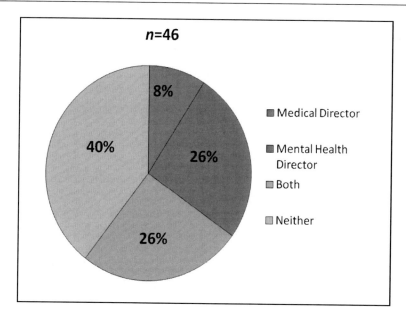

Figure 6. Medical and Mental Health Directors in State Child Welfare Agencies.

State child welfare agencies highlighted the need for access to up-to-date guidelines about mental health treatments, both psychosocial and psychotherapeutic among youth in child welfare custody. As one child welfare administrator noted, "Most children who are on meds are also receiving therapy, however the therapy may not be all that specific...we are not looking at other interventions enough." In particular, up-to-date information was needed across stakeholder groups including youth, caregivers, child welfare workers and administrators, prescribers, and other youth-serving organizations (e.g., schools, residential facilities). Respondents also cited the specific challenge that caregivers and child welfare workers confront when trying to express concern around particular treatment decisions to mental health providers; power differentials and limited mental health expertise may prohibit the caregiver or child welfare worker from asking questions necessary to be informed caregivers, advocates and/or decision-makers. As one child welfare administrator stated, "How do you educate your staff about psychotropic medications? Our caseworkers are not nurses or medical professionals, so how do you gear training?"

Practice Implications

Approaches states had taken to access mental health expertise and training on up-to-date guidelines included:

- Hiring staff or working with co-located Medicaid or mental health staff with mental health expertise within the child welfare system.
- Consulting with pediatric and mental health experts with expertise in treating children in child welfare custody. These experts may include clinicians at a local community public health department or mental health agency, or researchers at an academic medical center with interests in children in child welfare custody, public mental health, psychotropic medications, psychosocial interventions for behavior problems, or healthcare economics.

- Developing tele-psychiatry programs to address shortages of specialists in rural areas.
- Identifying reliable, up-to-date sources of information about clinical care, both for psychosocial and psychopharmacologic treatments, for children in child welfare custody (see Figure 7 for additional details).
- Providing clear guidance to prescribers about standards of care using AACAP guidelines/practice parameters and other resources.

Sponsor/Author	Publication
NIMH	Mental Health Medications (NIMH, 2012)
NIMH	Treatment of Children with Mental Illness (NIMH, 2009)
NIMH	Treatment of Children with Mental Disorders (NIMH, 2000)
NAMI	NAMI Policy Research Institute Task Force Report: Children and Psychotropic Medications (Gruttadaro and Miller, 2004)
AACAP	Psychiatric Medications for Children and Adolescents: Part I–How Medications Are Used (AACAP, 2004)
California Evidence-Based Clearinghouse	California Evidence-Based Clearinghouse Website (The California Evidence-Based Clearinghouse for Child Welfare, n.d.)

Note. AACAP = American Academy of Child and Adolescent Psychiatry; NAMI = National Alliance on Mental Illness; NIMH = National Institute of Mental Health.

Figure 7. Up-to-Date Guidelines: Examples.

Multi-Stakeholder Collaboration

Problem Statement

Child welfare agencies share responsibilities for the provision and payment of mental health services with other youth-serving systems. Medicaid, for example, is frequently the payer of mental health services for children in child welfare custody, while mental health departments may be critical to ensuring the provision of services. Partnerships with state Medicaid offices can be leveraged for prospective review of psychotropic medication requests (e.g., pre-authorization) or retrospective review of claims data that may be analyzed to determine diagnostic trends, types of treatments provided, and frequency of treatments. State level mental health administrators can help develop and disseminate practice guidelines for providers within a state as well as provide training for the broad range of stakeholders that are needed to help vulnerable children access and remain engaged in quality mental health care. Therefore, establishing systems to facilitate referral of children in child welfare custody to these other service delivery systems is often critical. A study conducted by Hurlburt and colleagues (2004) suggests that increased coordination between child welfare and mental health has been associated with additional mental healthcare utilization by children with the greatest level of need and with decreased racial/ethnic disparities in mental health service use. However, significant barriers may emerge in trying to coordinate service delivery between child welfare and other youth-serving systems (Allen, Hyde, and Leslie, 2012). Allen and colleagues (2012) found that differences in organizational culture and structure among youth-serving sectors (i.e., child welfare, public health, and early intervention) combined with inadequate fiscal, technological, and human resources, generated challenges in referring and serving children in child welfare custody.

Guidelines

While guidelines implicitly suggest the value of stakeholder collaboration to facilitate systems-development, relatively little is explicitly referenced. Only one of the guidelines reviewed explicitly identifies the importance of collaboration across youth-serving sectors; this guideline urges child welfare agencies to partner with the mental health sector (Romanelli et al., 2009). However, other guidelines implicitly refer to the need for collaboration in order to build upon resources offered by other youth-serving public systems. For example, guidelines emphasize the potential use of Medicaid's EPSDT funding as a vehicle to obtain mental health screens or the use of claims data to monitor psychotropic medication use (AACAP, 2011; AACAP and CWLA, 2003; AAP, District II New York State, Task Force on Health Care for Children in Foster Care, 2005) Yet, another guideline references the use of Medicaid claims data to inform child- and population-level monitoring systems (AACAP, 2011). None of the guidelines reviewed explicitly reference the involvement of child and family voices at the level of systems-development although this is inferred in calls for additional youth empowerment, family-centeredness, and family involvement in staffing structures (AACAP and CWLA, 2003; Jensen et al., 2009).

Study Findings

Most respondents voiced the critical importance of bringing together all involved stakeholders to develop a shared vision about the need for psychotropic medication oversight and to collaborate to implement that vision. One child welfare administrator stated, "No one agency can do it all – it must be a collaboration between social services, mental health, public health, and Medicaid." Many respondents commented on the lack of collaboration across state agencies, professionals, and organizations working with children in child welfare custody and how this hindered efforts to improve mental health care for these children. Some respondents noted that their states had neglected to include all stakeholders and found that this limited their success in achieving feasible and sustainable plans for mental health oversight. In addition, respondents emphasized the value of engaging mental health providers at the systems-development level (see Figure 6).

Practice Implications

States employed the following approaches to facilitate multi-stakeholder collaboration included:

- Recognizing that a mental health initiative for children in child welfare custody required a multi-system process and developed collaborative efforts with other state agencies (e.g., mental health, Medicaid, mental retardation/developmental delay, education, juvenile justice), and professional organizations (e.g., AAP, AACAP).
- Partnering with Medicaid or mental health to assist in monitoring psychotropic medication use among youth in child welfare custody. Examples include co-locating Medicaid or mental health staff with child welfare workers or having Medicaid or mental health staff provide feedback to "outliers."

- Developing a referral network of primary care and mental health clinicians with expertise in foster care.
- Establishing placement specialists in child welfare to work with foster parents around behaviors that result in placement changes.

CONCLUSION

Child welfare agencies have historically been concerned with the safety and protection of vulnerable children and families. Although children's well-being has long been a part of the mission of many child welfare agencies, what this means in policy and practice has, until late, not been well defined. This chapter has provided an overview of one indicator of well-being for children in child welfare custody – mental health - which has received increasing attention over the last decade. The move over the last few years by the Federal government to use policy mandates as a strategy to prioritize well-being generally, and mental health care specifically, has had a number of positive effects. In addition to heightened attention to the mental health care needs of children in child welfare custody, policy mandates also require that all states have plans in place to assure access to appropriate evaluation, treatment, and monitoring.

Assuring consistent access to the right mental health services begins with reliable screening and evaluation practices. These practices extend beyond an assessment tool to include engagement of youth, families and caregivers in conversations about concerning behaviors and experiences. Similarly, the movement from assessment to treatment requires both available resources and good communication between the many different people that may be responsible for children in child welfare custody. Strong, committed leadership from all levels of government will be needed in order for states to truly meet the mental health care needs of children in their care.

While intended to improve mental health outcomes for a population of children who are disproportionately affected by trauma and other adverse events, the movement from policy development to practice is not a formulaic or easy one. States' efforts to develop policies and practices to meet the mental health needs of children in child welfare custody have been challenged by a host of factors. In this chapter, we called attention to the limited resources (financial and human) available for quality mental health oversight, a lack of consensus among mental health providers regarding appropriate treatments for common mental health conditions among children with histories of trauma, difficulties in accessing real-time data to ensure compliance with state policies and practice guidelines, and the need to engage and improve the mental health literacy of children and families. The recent development of best practice guidelines, peer-reviewed articles and technical reports by a number of professional organizations have helped states identify what elements to include in their oversight plans and how to overcome some of the many challenges they face as they move from policy to practice.

The practice guidelines presented in this chapter highlight the multi-disciplinary effort that it will take to assure that policies are effectively and consistently implemented. Many states have already engaged partners from other state agencies, such as Medicaid, mental health, and public health, all of whom have specific expertise with some element of an oversight plan. What is clear from the guidance that is coming out from the Federal government and professional organizations is that child welfare administrators simply cannot meet the complex challenges of assuring mental health care for children in isolation. Strategic partnerships and innovative collaborations will be needed. Children in child welfare custody need and deserve the best mental health services that a state can provide. Strong committed leadership from multiple levels of government is necessary in order for states to truly meet the mental health care needs of children in their care.

ACKNOWLEDGMENTS

We would like to extend our appreciation to study respondents in state child welfare agencies across the United States. Throughout this work, we were deeply impressed with their commitment to meet the multiple needs of children and adolescents in child welfare custody. We are also appreciative of the assistance from our colleagues and research team at Tufts Medical Center; we are especially thankful for the collegial support and ongoing assistance of Jennifer Bakan, Christopher Bellonci, Emily H. Dawson, Carolyn Leung, Angie M. Rodday, and Tully Saunders.

Funding for this research was provided by grants from the Charles H. Hood Foundation and the W.T. Grant Foundation. The content of this paper is solely the responsibility of the authors and does not necessarily represent the views of our colleagues or the funding agencies listed above.

REFERENCES

Adoption and Safe Families Act of 1997, Pub. L. No. 105-89, 42 U.S.C. § 1305 (1997).

Aarons, G. A., and Palinkas, L. A. (2007). Implementation of evidence-based practice in child welfare: Service provider perspectives. *Administration and Policy in Mental Health and Mental Health Services Research, 34,* 411-419.

Allen, A. D., Hyde, J., and Leslie, L. K. (2012). "I don't know what they know:" Knowledge transfer in mandated referral from child welfare to early intervention. *Children and Youth Services Review, Advance online publication.* Epub ahead of print 21 Feb 2012.

American Academy of Child and Adolescent Psychiatry (2001). *AACAP policy statement on psychiatric care of children in the foster care system.* Retrieved from http://www. aacap.org/cs/root/policy_statements/psychiatric_care_of_children_in_the_foster_care_s ystem

American Academy of Child and Adolescent Psychiatry (2004). *Facts for families: Psychiatric medication for children and adolescents: Part 1 - How medications are used* (Report No. 21). Washington, DC. Retrieved from http://www.aacap.org /galleries/FactsForFamilies/21_psychiatric_medication_for_children_and_adolescents_ part_one.pdf

American Academy of Child and Adolescent Psychiatry (2009). Practice parameter on the use of psychotropic medication in children and adolescents. *Journal of the American Academy of Child and Adolescent Psychiatry, 48,* 961-973.

American Academy of Child and Adolescent Psychiatry (2011). *AACAP position statement on oversight of psychotropic medication use for children in state custody: A best principles guideline.* Retrieved from http://www.aacap.org/galleries/ Practice Information/FosterCare_BestPrinciples_FINAL.pdf.

American Academy of Child and Adolescent Psychiatry, and Child Welfare League of America (2003). *AACAP/CWLA policy statement on mental health and use of alcohol and other drugs, screening and assessment of children in foster care.* Retrieved from http://www.aacap.org/cs/root/policy_statements/aacap/cwla_policy_statement_on_ment al_health_and_use_of_alcohol_and_other_drugs_screening_and_assessment_of_childre n_in_foster_care.

American Academy of Pediatrics, Committee on Early Childhood, Adoption, and Dependent Care (2000). Developmental issues for young children in foster care. *Pediatrics, 106,* 1145-1150.

American Academy of Pediatrics, Committee on Early Childhood, Adoption, and Dependent Care (2002). Health care of young children in foster care. *Pediatrics, 109,* 536-541.

American Academy of Pediatrics, District II New York State, Task Force on Health Care for Children in Foster Care (2005). *Fostering health: Health care for children and adolescents in foster care* (2nd ed.). American Academy of Pediatrics.

Battistelli, E. S. (1996). *Making managed health care work for kids in foster care: A guide to purchasing services.* Washington, DC: CWLA Press.

Burns, B. J., Phillips, S. D., Wagner, H. R., Barth, R. P., Kolko, D. J., Campbell, Y. et al. (2004). Mental health need and access to mental health services by youths involved with child welfare: A national survey. *Journal of the American Academy of Child and Adolescent Psychiatry, 43,* 960-970.

Chaffin, M., and Friedrich, B. (2004). Evidence-based treatments in child abuse and neglect. *Children and Youth Services Review, 26,* 1097-1113.

Chernoff, R., Combs-Orme, T., Risley-Curtiss, C., and Heisler, A. (1994). Assessing the health status of children entering foster care. *Pediatrics, 93,* 594-601.

Child and Family Services Improvement and Innovation Act, Pub L. No. 112-34, 42 U.S.C. § 1305 (2011).

Child Welfare Information Gateway (2011). *Foster care statistics 2009.* Washington, DC: U.S. Department of Health and Human Services, Children's Bureau. Retrieved from http://www.childwelfare.gov/pubs/ factsheets/foster.cfm.

Child Welfare Information Gateway, Children's Bureau, Administration for Children and Families, U.S. Department of Health and Human Services (n.d). *Child welfare information gateway.* Retrieved from http://www.childwelfare.gov/

Clausen, J. M., Landsverk, J., Ganger, W., Chadwick, D., and Litrownik, A. (1998). Mental health problems of children in foster care. *Journal of Child and Family Studies, 7,* 283-296.

Courtney, M. E., and Dworsky, A. (2006). Early outcomes for young adults transitioning from outof-home care in the USA. *Child and Family Social Work, 11,* 209-219.

Courtney, M. E., Piliavin, I., Grogan-Kaylor, A., and Nesmith, A. (2001). Foster youth transitions to adulthood: A longitudinal view of youth leaving care. *Child Welfare, 80,* 685-717.

Courtney, M. E. and Wong, Y. L. I. (1996). Comparing the timing of exits from substitute care. *Children and Youth Services Review, 18,* 307-334.

Davies, J., and Wright, J. (2008). Children's voices: A review of the literature pertinent to looked-after children's views of mental health services. *Child and Adolescent Mental Health, 13*, 26-31.

Dore, M. (2005). Child and adolescent mental health. In G. P. Mallon and P. Hess (Eds.), *Child welfare for the twenty-first century: A handbook of practices, policies, and programs (2nd ed.)* (pp. 148-172). New York, NY: Columbia University Press.

dosReis, S., Zito, J. M., Safer, D. J., and Soeken, K. L. (2001). Mental health services for youths in foster care and disabled youths. *American Journal of Public Health, 91*, 1094-1099.

Ferguson, D. G., Glesener, D. C., and Raschick, M. (2006). Psychotropic drug use with European American and American Indian children in foster care. *Journal of Child and Adolescent Psychopharmacology, 16*, 474-481.

Fostering Connections to Success and Increasing Adoptions Act of 2008, Pub L. No. 110-351, 42 U.S.C. § 1305 (2008).

Garland, A. F., Hough, R. L., Landsverk, J. A., and Brown, S. A. (2001). Multi-sector complexity of systems of care for youth with mental health needs. *Children's Services: Social Policy, Research, and Practice, 4*, 123-140.

Garland, A. F., Hough, R. L., Landsverk, J. A., McCabe, K. M., Yeh, M., Ganger, W. C. et al. (2000). Racial and ethnic variations in mental health care utilization among children in foster care. *Children's services: Social Policy, Research, and Practice, 3*, 133-146.

Garland, A. F., Landsverk, J. L., Hough, R. L., and Ellis-Macleod, E. (1996). Type of maltreatment as a predictor of mental health service use for children in foster care. *Child Abuse and Neglect, 20*, 675-688.

Goodwin, R., Gould, M. S., Blanco, C., and Olfson, M. (2001). Prescription of psychotropic medications to youths in office-based practice. *Psychiatric Services, 52*, 1081-1087.

Government Accountability Office (2011). *HHS guidance could help states improve oversight of psychotropic prescriptions* (Rep. No. GAO-12-270T). Washington, DC: United States Government Accountability Office. Retrieved from http://www.gao.gov/ products/GAO-12-270T.

Gruttadaro, D. E. and Miller, J. E. (2004). *NAMI Policy Research Institute Task Force Report: Children and psychotropic medications.* Arlington, VA: National Alliance on Mental Illness. Retrieved from http://www.nami.org/ Template.cfm?Section=Research_ Services_and_Treatmentandtemplate=/ContentManagement/ContentDisplay.cfmandCo ntentID=38449.

Halfon, N. and Klee, L. (1987). Health services for California's foster children: current practices and policy recommendations. *Pediatrics, 80*, 183-191.

Hockstadt, N. J., Jaudes, P. K., Zimo, D. A., and Schachter, J. (1987). The medical and psychosocial needs of children entering foster care. *Child Abuse and Neglect, 11*, 53-62.

Horwitz, S. M., Chamberlain, P., Landsverk, J., and Mullican, C. (2010). Improving the mental health of children in child welfare through the implementation of evidence-based parenting interventions. *Administration and Policy in Mental Health and Mental Health Services Research, 37*, 27-39.

Horwitz, S. M., Simms, M. D., and Farrington, R. (1994). Impact of developmental problems on young children's exits from foster care. *Journal of Developmental and Behavioral Pediatrics, 15*, 105-110.

Hurlburt, M. S., Leslie, L. K., Landsverk, J., Barth, R. P., Burns, B. J., Gibbons, R. D. et al. (2004). Contextual predictors of mental health service use among children open to child welfare. *Archives of General Psychiatry, 61,* 1217-1224.

Iglehart, J. K. (2003). The dilemma of Medicaid. *The New England Journal of Medicine, 348,* 2140-2148.

Jensen, P. J., Romanelli, L. H., Pecora, P. J., and Ortiz, A. (2009). Special issue: Mental health practice guidelines reform. *Child Welfare, 88(1).*

Jorm, A. F. (2000). Mental health literacy: Public knowledge and beliefs about mental disorders. *British Journal of Psychiatry, 177,* 396-401.

Kansas Health Policy Authority (2009). *2008 Medicaid Transformation: Kansas Medicaid Program Reviews Plan.* Topeka: KS: Kansas Department of Health and Environment. Retrieved from http://www.kdheks.gov/hcf/medicaid_transformation/download/2008/KHPA_2008_Medicaid_Transformation.pdf.

Kaplan, S. J., Skolnik, L., and Turnbull, A. (2009). Enhancing the empowerment of youth in foster care: Supportive services. *Child Welfare, 88,* 133-161.

Kavaler, F., and Swire, M. R. (1983). *Foster-child health care.* Lexington, MA: Lexington Books.

Kolko, D. J., Hurlburt, M. S., Zhang, J., Barth, R. P., Leslie, L. K., and Burns, B. J. (2010). Posttraumatic stress symptoms in children and adolescents referred for child welfare investigation: A national sample of in-home and out-of-home care. *Child Maltreatment, 15,* 48-63.

Kolko, D. J., Selelyo, J., and Brown, E. J. (1999). The treatment histories and service involvement of physically and sexually abusive families: Description, correspondence, and clinical correlates. *Child Abuse and Neglect, 23,* 459-476.

Kupsinel, M. M., and Dubsky, D. D. (1999). Behaviorally impaired children in out-of-home care. *Child Welfare, 78,* 297-310.

Landsverk, J., Davis, I., Ganger, W., Newton, R., and Johnson, I. (1996). Impact of child psychosocial functioning on reunification from out-of-home placement. *Children and Youth Services Review, 18,* 447-462.

Landsverk, J., Garland, A. F., and Leslie, L. K. (2002). Mental health services for children reported to child protective services. In J. E. B. Myers, L. Berliner, J. Briere, C. T. Hendrix, C. Jenny, and T. A. Reid (Eds.), *ASPAC Handbook on Child Maltreatment (2nd ed.)* (pp. 467-507). Thousand Oaks, CA: Sage Publications.

Landsverk, J. A., Burns, B. J., Stambaugh, L. F., and Rolls-Reutz, J. A. (2006). *Mental health care for children and adolescents in foster care: Review of research literature.e* Seattle, WA: Case Family Programs.

Leslie, L. K., Gordon, J. N., Lambros, K., Premji, K., Peoples, J., and Gist, K. (2005a). Addressing the developmental and mental health needs of young children in foster care. *Journal of Developmental and Behavioral Pediatrics, 26,* 140-151.

Leslie, L. K., Hurlburt, M. S., James, S., Landsverk, J., Slymen, D. J., and Zhang, J. (2005b). Relationship between entry into child welfare and mental health service use. *Psychiatric Services, 56,* 981-987.

Leslie, L. K., Hurlburt, M. S., Landsverk, J., Barth, R., and Slymen, D. J. (2004). Outpatient mental health services for children in foster care: A national perspective. *Child Abuse and Neglect, 28,* 699-714.

Leslie, L. K., Hurlburt, M. S., Landsverk, J., Rolls, J. A., Wood, P. A., and Kelleher, K. J. (2003a). Comprehensive assessments for children entering foster care: A national perspective. *Pediatrics, 112,* 134-142.

Leslie, L. K., Kelleher, K. J., Burns, B. J., Landsverk, J., and Rolls, J. A. (2003b). Foster care and Medicaid managed care. *Child Welfare, 82,* 367-392.

Leslie, L. K., Landsverk, J., Ezzet-Lofstrom, R., Tschann, J. M., Slymen, D. J., and Garland, A. F. (2000). Children in foster care: Factors influencing outpatient mental health service use. *Child Abuse and Neglect, 24,* 465-476.

Leslie, L. K., Mackie, T. I., Dawson, E. H., Bellonci, C., Schoonover, D. R., Rodday, A. M. et al. (2010). *Multi-state study on psychotropic medication oversight in foster care. Study report and appendix.* Boston, MA: Tufts University Clinical and Translational Science Institute.

Leslie, L. K., Mackie, T. I., Mulé, C., Wade, R., Rubin, C. L., Dawson, E. H. et al. (2011). *Examination of the Rogers process for youth in the custody of the Massachusetts Department of Children and Families. Study report and appendix.* Boston, MA: Tufts University Clinical and Translational Science Institute.

Leslie, L. K., Raghavan, R., Zhang, J., and Aarons, G. A. (2010). Rates of psychotropic medication use over time among youth in child welfare/child protective services. *Journal of Child and Adolescent Psychopharmacology, 20,* 135-143.

Littner, N. (1956). *Some traumatic effects of separation and placement.* New York, NY: Child Welfare League of America.

Mackie, T. I., Hyde, J., Rodday, A. M., Dawson, E., Lakshmikanthan, R., Bellonci, C. et al. (2011). Psychotropic medication oversight for youth in foster care: A national perspective on state child welfare policy and practice guidelines. *Children and Youth Services Review, 33,* 2213-2220.

McMillen, J. C., and Tucker, J. (1999). The status of older adolescents at exit from out-of-home care. *Child Welfare, 78,* 339-362.

McMillen, J. C., Zima, B. T., Scott Jr, L. D., Auslander, W. F., Munson, M. R., Ollie, M. T. et al. (2005). Prevalence of psychiatric disorders among older youths in the foster care system. *Journal of the American Academy of Child and Adolescent Psychiatry, 44,* 88-95.

National Institute of Mental Health (2000). *Treatment of children with mental disorders* (NIH Publication No. 00-470). Bethesda, MD: National Institute of Mental Health, National Institutes of Health, U.S. Department of Health and Human Services. Retrieved from http://wwwapps.nimh. nih.gov/health/publications/treatment-of-children-with-mental-disorders/ complete.pdf.

National Institute of Mental Health (2009). *Treatment of children with mental illness: Frequently asked questions about the treatment of mental illness in children* (NIH Publication No. 09-470). Bethesda, MD: National Institute of Mental Health, National Institutes of Health, U.S. Department of Health and Human Services. Retrieved from http://www.nimh.nih.gov/health/publications/treatment-of-children-with-mental-illness-fact-sheet/nimh-treatment-children-mental-illness-faq.pdf.

National Institute of Mental Health (2012). *Mental health medications* (NIH Publication No. 12–3929). Bethesda, MA: National Institute of Mental Health, National Institutes of Health, U.S. Department of Health and Human Services. Retrieved from http://www.

nimh.nih.gov/health/publications/mental-health-medications/nimh-mental-health-medications. pdf.

National Resource Center for Permanency and Family Connections (2012). *Handbooks and resources for children and youth in foster care.* Retrieved from http://www. hunter.cuny.edu/socwork/nrcfcpp/info_services/ handbooks-for-youth.html.

Naylor, M. W., Davidson, C. V., Ortega-Piron, D. J., Bass, A., Gutierrez, A., and Hall, A. (2007). Psychotropic medication management for youth in state care: consent, oversight, and policy considerations. *Child Welfare, 86,* 175-192.

Newton, R. R., Litrownik, A. J., and Landsverk, J. A. (2000). Children and youth in foster care: Disentangling the relationship between problem behaviors and number of placements. *Child Abuse and Neglect, 24,* 1363-1374.

Olfson, M., Blanco, C., Liu, L. X., Moreno, C., and Laje, G. (2006). National trends in the outpatient treatment of children and adolescents with antipsychotic drugs. *Archives of General Psychiatry, 63,* 679-685.

Olfson, M., Gameroff, M. J., Marcus, S. C., and Waslick, B. D. (2003). Outpatient treatment of child and adolescent depression in the United States. *Archives of General Psychiatry, 60,* 1236-1242.

Olfson, M., Marcus, S. C., Weissman, M. M., and Jensen, P. S. (2002). National trends in the use of psychotropic medications by children. *Journal of the American Academy of Child and Adolescent Psychiatry, 41,* 514-521.

Pecora, P. J., Williams, J., Kessler, R. C., Downs, A. C., O'Brien, K., Hiripi, E. et al. (2003). *Assessing the effects of foster care: Early results from the Casey National Alumni Study.* Seattle, WA: Casey Family Programs. Retrieved from http://www. inpathways. net/casey_alumni_studies_ report.pdf

Pilowsky, D. (1995). Psychopathology among children placed in family foster care. *Psychiatric Services, 46,* 906-910.

Raghavan, R., Bright, C. L., and Shadoin, A. L. (2008). Toward a policy ecology of implementation of evidence-based practices in public mental health settings. *Implementation Science, 3,* 26.

Rickwood, D., Deane, F. P., Wilson, C. J., and Ciarrochi, J. (2005). Young people's help-seeking for mental health problems. *Advances in Mental Health, 4,* 218-251.

Romanelli, L. H., Landsverk, J., Levitt, J. M., Leslie, L. K., Hurley, M. M., Bellonci, C. et al. (2009). Best practices for mental health in child welfare: Screening, assessment, and treatment guidelines. *Child welfare, 88,* 163-188.

Schor, E. L. (1982). The foster care system and health status of foster children. *Pediatrics, 69,* 521-528.

Schor, E. L. (1988). Foster care. *Pediatric Clinics of North America, 35,* 1241-1252.

Simms, M. D., and Kelly, R. W. (1991). Pediatricians and foster children. *Child Welfare, 70,* 451-461.

Stahmer, A. C., Leslie, L. K., Hurlburt, M., Barth, R. P., Webb, M. B., Landsverk, J. et al. (2005). Developmental and behavioral needs and service use for young children in child welfare. *Pediatrics, 116,* 891-900.

Strayhorn, C. K. (2006). *Texas health care claims study - special report on foster children.* Austin: TX: Office of the Comptroller, Texas Comptroller of Public Accounts. Retrieved from http://psychrights.org/states/Texas/ hccfoster06.pdf.

The California Evidence-Based Clearinghouse for Child Welfare (n.d). *California evidence-based clearinghouse for child welfare*. Retrieved from http://www.cebc4cw.org.

U.S. Department of Health and Human Services, Administration for Children and Families, Administration on Children, Youth and Families, Children's Bureau (2011). *Child maltreatment 2010*. Retrieved from http://www. acf.hhs.gov/programs/cb/stats_ research/index.htm#can.

U.S. Department of Health and Human Services, Administration for Children and Families, Administration on Children, Youth and Families, Children's Bureau (2011). *The AFCARS report: Preliminary estimates for FY 2010 as of June 2011* (Rep. No. 18). Retrieved from http://www. acf.hhs.gov/programs/cb/stats_research/afcars/tar /report 18.pdf.

Wulczyn, F., Barth, R. P., Yuan, Y. T., Harden, B. J., and Landsverk, J. (2005). *Beyond common sense: Child welfare, child well-being, and the evidence for policy reform*. Piscataway, NJ: Aldine Transaction.

Yudkowsky, B. K., Cartland, J. D., and Flint, S. S. (1990). Pediatrician participation in Medicaid: 1978 to 1989. *Pediatrics, 85*, 567-577.

Zito, J. M., Safer, D. J., Sai, D., Gardner, J. F., Thomas, D., Coombes, P. et al. (2008). Psychotropic medication patterns among youth in foster care. *Pediatrics, 121*, e157-e163.

In: Child Welfare
Editors: Alex Powell and Jenna Gray-Peterson

ISBN: 978-1-62257-826-9
© 2013 Nova Science Publishers, Inc.

Chapter 2

CHILDREN IN FOSTER CARE
AND EXCESSIVE MEDICATIONS

Jill Littrrell[*]

Georgia State University, School of Social Work, Atlanta, Georgia, US

ABSTRACT

Children in foster care system are more likely to receive diagnoses of major mental illness and to be medicated with powerful medications such as antipsychotic drugs. Reasons for the increased risk of the actual mental illnesses and for the diagnoses of illness among children in foster care are reviewed. The reliabilities of various diagnoses are considered. The legitimacy of the rationale for early medications to prevent later disability is discussed. The very real hazards of medicating with antipsychotics, anticonvulsants, stimulants, mood stabilizers and antidepressants are reviewed. A discussion of advocacy efforts occurring around the United States on behalf of medicated children in the foster care system is presented. Finally, changes being instituted by the federal government through the Department of Health, Education, and Welfare and the Government Accounting Office (GAO), following the hearing of December 1, 2011 convened by Senator Thomas Carper, are discussed.

CHILDREN IN FOSTER CARE: A VULNERABLE POPULATION

Medicating Foster Children

In the last decade, the use of antipsychotic medications for adults and children has increased dramatically. Domino and Swartz (2008) compared prescriptions for antipsychotic medications in 1996-1997 with prescriptions for antipsychotics in 2004-2005. The rate of adult office visits resulting in antipsychotics rose from 0.6% to 1.3% while the rate for children rose from 0.2% to 0.7%. Moreover, Comer, Mojtabai, and Olfson (2011)

---

[*] Littrell@gsu.edu

documented the recent rise in the use of atypical antipsychotics to treat anxiety disorders. Antipsychotics are also currently being used to treat antidepressant resistant depression and ADHD (Crystal, Olfson, Huang, Pincus, Gerhard, 2009; Fullerton et al., 2011) and insomnia (Sinaikin, 2010). The increase is especially large among children in foster care. A study of 16 state Medicaid programs in 2007 found that 1.6% of children younger than 19 were receiving antipsychotics while 12.37% of children in foster care were receiving antipsychotics (Medicaid Medical Directors Leaning Network, 2010, p. 14). dosReis et al. (2011) examined psychotropic prescriptions for 16,969 children under 20 years of age in a Mid-Atlantic state Medicaid program. All of the children in the sample had been given a mental health diagnoses. For the children in foster care not awaiting adoption, 19% were being medicated with multiple antipsychotic drugs and 24% of children who were in foster care awaiting adoption were being treated with multiple antipsychotics. Similar patterns of greater use of psychotropic drugs of many classes were found in a number of additional studies comparing rates of medicating foster children to other children (Breland-Noble et al., 2004; DosReis et al., 2001; Raghavan et al., 2005; Raghavan and McMillen, 2008).

Most recently, on December 1, 2011, Senator Tom Carper held a hearing to discuss the Government Accounting Office's study of the psychiatric treatment of children in foster care. The Government Accounting Office (Kutz, 2011) issued a report on the medication of children in foster care in five states during 2008. Across states, children in foster care are 2.7 to 4.5 times more likely to be medicated than children receiving Medicaid. Infants younger than 1 are medicated, albeit possibly with Benadryl (Salo, 2011). Doses exceeding the maximum levels approved by the FDA were found in several states. Across states, 0.11 to 1.33 percent of children are being treated concurrently with over five medications. According to the GAO panel "our experts also said that no evidence supports the use of five or more psychotropic drugs in adults or children, and only limited evidence supports the use of even two drugs concomitantly in children (Kutz, 2011, p14)."

Increased Risk for Mental Illness in Children in Foster Care

Greater prevalence of a number of mental illnesses might be expected in a population of foster children. First, many mental illnesses have a hereditary component. Parental mental disorder may constitute the reason why a child is in foster care. Because a child shares hereditary risk with a parent, greater prevalence of particular disorders can be expected for children in foster care. Second, disorders such as major depression, PTSD, and anxiety disorders are exacerbated by stressful conditions. The National Survey of Child and Adolescent Well-Being finds that 70% of children in foster care have a history of child abuse and/or neglect, more than 80% had biological parents with impaired parenting skills, and 40% had witnessed domestic violence (Burns et al., 2004; Leslie, Kelleher, Burns, Landsverk, and Rolls, 2003; Stahmer et al., 2005). Once in the foster care system, 63% of foster children are placed out of home for a duration of less than two years and during those two years live in, on average, three different placements (US DHHS, 2007). Thus, stressful conditions prior in early life and unstable living situations once in the foster care system can be expected to exacerbate emotional problems. Third, loss of a biological parent alone can be expected to result in depressive and anxiety symptoms as well as Post Traumatic Stress Disorder (PTSD) in children.

Indeed, the GAO (2011) report noted that "57% of foster children were diagnosed with a mental disorder—nearly 15 times that of non-foster children receiving Medicaid assistance."

Issue of Legitimacy of Diagnosis

In an earlier time making a correct diagnosis was important because diagnosis was a guide to selecting the proper treatment. However, as previously documented, currently major depression, ADHD, anxiety disorders, and sleep disorders are being treated with atypical antipsychotics. DosReis et al. (2011) found that of the foster children in their sample receiving an antipsychotic, 53% had a diagnosis of ADHD, 34% had a diagnosis of depression, 21% had a diagnosis of bipolar, while only 5% had a diagnosis of schizophrenia. In examining factors that contributed to the greater likelihood of receiving multiple antipsychotics concomitantly, being male, being African American, and having diagnoses of conduct disorder, autism, bipolar, psychosis, and schizophrenia increased the probability. Many of the children in the sample being treated with antipsychotics were also receiving antidepressants, stimulants, and mood stabilizers. In current practice, correspondence between diagnoses and particular treatments no longer describes practice. DosReis et al. (2011) speculated regarding the rationale for using multiple antipsychotics concurrently. They suggested that an insufficient response to one drug might prompt the addition of a second drug rather than increasing the dosage of the first drug or, perhaps, adding a second drug for a sleep problem might have provided a rationale. They also considered that "a proportion might lack a reasonable clinical rationale (p.1464")". Whatever the reason, antipsychotics seem to be being dispensed for a wide range of diagnoses.

While individual physicians are engaging in off-label use of various drugs such as antipsychotics for various diagnoses in children and adults, the Federal Drug Administration continues to approve drugs for particular diagnoses rather than as general purpose panaceas. Assuming that diagnoses are still relevant in clinical practice, two diagnostic categories, which are not in the DSM-IV-R but have gained a modicum of perceived legitimacy, will be discussed: Pediatric Bipolar and Pre-psychosis.

Pediatric Bipolar

Before the last decade, there was wide agreement that Bipolar Disorder did not emerge prior to late adolescence or young adulthood (Anthony and Scott, 1960; Goodwin and Jamison, 2007, p. 188; Loranger and Levine, 1978). Whereas in 1996, pediatric bipolar was the least frequent diagnosis in hospitalized children, by 2004, it was the most frequent diagnosis for hospitalized children (Blader and Carlson, 2007). How did the diagnosis of Pediatric Bipolar gain acceptance? In the 1990s, Joseph Biederman, a child psychiatrist at Harvard, and his colleagues, began publishing articles indicating that many of the children who were being diagnosed as having ADHD and/or conduct disorder, also met criteria for Bipolar Disorder (see Biederman, Mick, Faraone, Spencer, Wilens, and Wozniak, 2000; Biederman et al., 2003).

In order to bolster his case for children actually having Bipolar disorder, Biederman and colleagues and others assessed the parents of those children who met criteria for Bipolar disorder (see review of studies in Littrell and Lyons, 2010a). Many of these parents also met criteria for Bipolar Spectrum diagnoses.

Since Bipolar is widely accepted as a heritable disease, the findings in parents were purported as evidence for the legitimacy of the claim that these children really were bipolar and they would emerge as adults with Bipolar Disorder.

Flaws in the Argument

Biederman was able to make the case that the parents of the children who were being diagnosed with bipolar were also bipolar because of changes in the DSM-IV. In 1994, the diagnosis of Bipolar II was added to the *Diagnostic and Statistical Manual-IV* of the American Psychiatric Association. In in the 1994 manual and the current 2000 version of the manual, whereas a diagnosis of Bipolar I requires that a patient meet criteria for an episode of mania, a diagnosis of Bipolar II only requires meeting criteria for hypomania. The same behaviors are listed for both mania and hypomania.

The difference is that mania must last for a week whereas only four days are required for hypomania and most importantly, if the behaviors result in functional impairment, then the diagnosis of mania is given rather than hypomania (see DSM-IV-TR, 2000, p. 368). The fact that hypomania does not result in significant functional impairment (DSM-IV-R) and the fact that hypomania is very common in the general population (Udachina and Mansell, 2007; Wicki and Angst, 1991) augured that the diagnosis of Bipolar would sky-rocket. Indeed, Moreno, Laje, Blanco, Jiang, Schmidt, and Olfson (2007) have documented a 38% increase in adult bipolar diagnoses from 2002-2003 compared to 1994-1995.

The problem with the diagnoses of Bipolar I and Bipolar II is they are two distinct disorders. In an early study, tracking those with Bipolar II diagnoses over time found that they were very unlikely to meet criteria for mania in later life (Coryell et al., 1995). Studies examining the family members of those with Bipolar I and Bipolar II, established that relatives of those with Bipolar I, for the most part, met criteria for Bipolar I and relatives of those with Bipolar II, for the most part, met criteria for Bipolar II (e.g., Coryell et al., 1984; see Littrell and Lyons, 2010a for review).

The alleles for various genes increasing the risk for Bipolar I are not shared by those with Bipolar II (Judd et al., 2003; Vieta and Suppes, 2008). Moreover, distinct trajectories describe the course of the two disorders over time (Judd et al., 2003). Thus, the common label "bipolar" for those meeting criteria for Bipolar I and Bipolar II is very misleading. In the studies examining the parents of children with Pediatric Bipolar, researchers failed to distinguish whether the parents met criteria for Bipolar I or Bipolar II (Littrell and Lyons, 2010a). Thus, the inference that children meeting criteria for Pediatric Bipolar had a genetic predisposition for Bipolar Disorder I based on the findings from studies of their parents was not legitimate and very misleading.

There were additional reasons for questioning whether children being diagnosed as Pediatric Bipolar would ever become Bipolar I adults. Many retrospective studies of adults with well-characterized Bipolar I suggested that they had exhibited depressive symptoms but not mania symptoms as children.

For most adults with Bipolar I, a diagnosis of Major Depression preceded the emergence of mania. Moreover, there were a number of longitudinal studies of the children of parents with well characterized Bipolar I Disorder. Typical of these studies is work of Anne Duffy and colleagues. In a recent publication, Duffy, Alda, Hajek, and Grof (2009) reported that in their now young adult children of parents with Bipolar I, mania never emerged prior to 12, the mean age for the emergence of mania was 17, and in those in whom mania emerged, it was most often presaged by depressive symptoms in childhood. Thus, the children being diagnosed with Pediatric Bipolar, whose behavior overlapped with Attention Deficit/Hyperactivity, were obviously from a different population. (See Littrell and Lyons, 2010a, for citations and a review of the material referred to in this section.)

While psychiatrists are employing the Pediatric Bipolar diagnosis with great regularity, the various Committees established to develop diagnoses for children in the forthcoming DSM-V report are considering diagnoses of Temper Dysregulation Disorder with Dysphoria and Severe Mood Dysregulation (DSM-V Mood Disorders Workgroup; DSM-V Childhood and Adolescent Disorder Work Group, 2011) to supplant the Pediatric Bipolar label. Both antidepressants and stimulants can precipitate manic behavior (Delbello et al., 2001; Ghaemi, Hsu, Soldani, and Goodwin, 2003; Martin et al., 2004; Spetie and Arnold, 2007).

The workgroups have noted that alternative terminology, a mere change in wording, could reopen the question of appropriate treatment for children currently being labeled Pediatric Bipolar.

The committee recognized that for persons to whom the label "bipolar" is applied, "current convention renders treatment with antidepressants or stimulants relatively contraindicated without concurrent mood stabilizers or antipsychotics, (p. 6)." The discussions of the DSM-V workgroups reveal the degree to which confusion reigns as to how to identify legitimate diagnoses and what constitutes good treatment.

Pre-Psychosis

Considerable research has focused on the identification of markers that presage the development of psychosis. The hope was to be able to intervene early in the process and prevent schizophrenia. Allen Frances (2010b; 2011c), Co-Chair of the DSM-IV, articulates his objection to Pre-Psychosis in the forthcoming DSM-V. He argues that predictors of psychosis are not yet sensitive or specific. Indeed, Thompson, Nelson, and Yung (2011), developers of criteria for predicting future psychosis, reported that only 64.5% of those who developed schizophrenia were identified by their battery and for those scoring high, 35% were false positives.

Examining persons in the high risk category, only 39.4% transitioned to psychosis during the 28 month follow-up interval. Thus, even given the best tools for identifying persons who will become psychotic, false positives are high. Allen Frances argues that given the state of the art, labeling children as "pre-psychotic" would not only be stigmatizing but would also result in unneeded medications.

Post Traumatic Stress Disorder

Many of the symptoms exhibited by children in foster care who are being medicated overlap with symptoms of PTSD. Hyper-alertness, irritability, and emotionality have been noted in Veterans returning from Iraq (Tyre, 2004). Thus, behavioral disturbance can be expected in those suffering trauma. Certainly, all children in foster care meet criteria for trauma: all have been removed from their biological families.

Presently, reliable methods for distinguishing responses to trauma from other disorders in children have not been proffered. It is notable that the American Academy of Child and Adolescent Psychiatry (Gleason et al., 2007) specifically advises that PTSD in children should be treated with talk therapy and should not be medicated.

Can Early Pharmacological Intervention Change the Course of a Disorder?

Bipolar

Kiki Chang and colleagues (2010; Chang, Howe, Galleli, and Miklowitz, 2006; Chang and Kowatch, 2007) have been proponents of the idea that early pharmaceutical treatment of Bipolar Disorder can prevent the emergence of severe symptoms. For his rationale, Chang references the kindling theory proffered by Robert Post (2007). The kindling theory posits that some process occurs in the brain when individuals are symptomatic which alters the physical characteristics so that severe symptoms are easier to elicit afterwards. If symptoms can be blocked, the kindling process can be precluded and the brain will remain healthy. That is the theory. Do the data support the theory?

In his many publications Chang fails to acknowledge some relevant facts. First, Goodwin and Jamison (2007), in their classic work on Bipolar, find little evidence for the kindling hypothesis that greater initial symptoms play a causal role in creating later symptoms(see Goodwin and Jamison, 2007, p. 152). With regard to early treatment changing the course of the disorder, Baldessarinni and colleagues have examined the impact of early treatment on the course of the Bipolar disorder and conclude that early treatment has no impact on subsequent frequency or severity of mood episodes (Baethge et al., 2003; Baldessarini, Tondo, Baethge, and Bratti, 2007). Finally, in Post's research on kindling which involved inducing seizure activity in rodents, suppression of seizures with anticonvulsants did not alter later sensitivity to provoking seizures, in fact, lamotrigine and carbamazine facilitated kindling (Post, 2004; Weiss, Clark, Rosen, Smith, and Post, 1995; Postma, Krupp, Li, Post, and Weiss, 2000). Thus, the logic behind the rationale for early treatment is not supported by the facts. As we will be discussed in a later section, all of the drugs for Bipolar have severe deleterious effects on health. Thus, delaying treatment as long as possible seems a worthy goal.

While evidence is lacking for early treatment altering long term outcome, Whitaker (2010) has questioned whether pharmacological interventions for Bipolar I in adults, in fact, impairs long term outcome. Although drugs are approved by the FDA on the basis of evidence of efficacy, it should be noted that drug efficacy studies observe patients for about eight weeks. There have been no studies with random assignment to treatment and placebo with long term follow-up over years. An early naturalistic study with a ten year follow-up by Winokur et al. (1994) concluded that medications were not significantly related to outcome for patients with Bipolar.

Without the availability of random control studies to assess long term outcome of treatment, one can contrast the pre-drug literature on outcomes for Bipolar Disorder with current long term studies. This is what Whitaker did in his book. With regard to evaluation of patients before drugs, Rennie (1942) found that 93% of patients with mania recovered from their initial episode in an average of several months. Twenty-one percent never relapsed. Of those who did relapse, 30% remained remitted for at least 10 years with an average duration of remission of 20 years. Thus, after an initial period of bipolar symptoms, 51% were remaining well for a significant period of time. Later studies of those with Bipolar I in the post drug era find that only 2.1% of persons are asymptomatic during a 12.8 year follow-up; 80% of those who recover relapse within 1.7 years; 23% are continuously unemployed and another 35% are erratically employed (Harrow, Goldberg, Grossman, and Meltzer, 1990; Judd et al., 2002). Examining outcomes for those with Bipolar II, Judd et al. (2003) concluded that Bipolar II is an even more chronic condition than Bipolar I.

Psychiatrists have also provided global assessments of outcomes for Bipolar Disorder. A review of early studies prompted Winokur, Clayton, and Reich (1969) to conclude there "was no basis to consider manic depressive psychosis permanently affected those who suffered from it" (p.21). This contrasts with the dismal prognosis, provided by the Judd et al. (2002) findings in the longest follow-up study of medicated patients in the post-drug literature discussed previously. Zarate, Tohen, Land, and Cavanagh (2000) have also noted the contrast between earlier and current outcomes: "In the era prior to pharmacotherapy, poor outcome in mania was considered a relatively rare occurrence. However, modern outcome studies have found that a majority of bipolar patients evidence high rates of functional impairment" (p. 309). The contrast between early conclusions on Bipolar Disorder with current outcome studies should have prompted the hypothesis that drugs create a worse outcome. Rather, the conclusion made by psychiatrists is that in modern times we conduct more sensitive research and thus can develop more realistic expectations of prognosis.

It should be noted that the efficacy of lithium for reducing bipolar symptoms in children ages 7-17 has been called into question (Dickstein et al., 2008).

Pre-psychosis and Psychosis

In examining efficacy of early medicating of psychosis, two types of studies can be examined. The first literature considers studies asking whether early treatment for those exhibiting overt psychosis changes the long term outcome of the later course of psychosis. Most of the studies in this literature were on young adults and not children. Indeed, in a meta-analysis by Perkins et al. (2005), the mean age of those with first episode psychosis was 27.8, so direct relevance to children can be questioned. However, this literature does shed light on the effects of early treatment. Another set of studies has examined the impact of treatment intervention on those who only exhibit symptoms believed to be predictive of later psychosis and who may have relatives with psychosis. The issue of the efficacy of early treatment of those already exhibiting psychotic symptoms, for psychosis and the issue of preventing psychosis are examined separately.

Treating overt Psychosis Early

Two large meta-analysis (Marshall et al., 2005; Perkins, Gu, Boteva, and Lieberman, 2005) have concluded that in those individuals exhibiting delusional thinking or experiencing hallucinations, delaying treatment is associated with more negative outcome. However, both of these reviews identified significant caveats in drawing the conclusion that early treatment causes better outcome. In both the Perkins et al. and Marshall et al. reviews, those receiving delays in treatment were distinguished by greater negative symptoms. Some of the positive benefit of early treatment was attenuated after controlling for initial characteristics. Moreover, in both reviews difference in outcome between those receiving early and late treatment was modest, with Perkins noting that delay in treatment accounted for only 13% of the variance in outcome.

Preventing the Emergence of Psychosis

A number of investigators have evaluated interventions to reduce the transition to psychosis in samples selected for high risk. No clear benefit for psychotherapy, family interventions, or antipsychotic drugs was apparent according to a review conducted by the

Cocharane Collaboration (Marshall and Rathbone, 2011a, b). However, there was a suggestive positive result from the use of omega-3 fatty acid supplements. In a study by Amminger et al. (2010), 81 high risk subjects were randomly assigned to take omega-3s or placebo. They were evaluated on global functioning and level of symptoms at 52 weeks. Some of the patients in the omega-3 group and the control group were taking benzodiazepines or antidepressants but none were taking antipsychotics. By 52 weeks, 4.9% of the omega-3 group and 27.5% of the placebo group had transitioned to psychotic disorder (Amminger et al., 2010). Along with the just-cited suggestive evidence for efficacy of omega-3 in preventing the emergence of psychosis, there is evidence that omega-3 have strong antidepressant properties (Kiecolt-Glaser, 2010). Moreover, in a study of medical students, omega-3 supplementation did attenuate symptoms of stress (Kiecolt-Glaser, Belury, Andridge, Malarkey, and Glaser, 2011). Omega-3s are found in fish and walnuts. Dietary supplements are also available.

ADHD

Years ago, Judith Rappoport and colleagues (Sostek, Buchsbaum, and Rapoport, 1980) conducted a study in which she gave stimulants to all the children, both those with ADHD and those without. She found that attention and vigilance improved for all children administered the stimulant. Stimulants are noted for focusing attention and enhancing memory formation in adults (Hart, Ksir, and Ray, 2009; Soetens, D'Hooge, Huesting, 1993). Studies evaluating improvement in school performance, do find that children with ADHD do better with stimulants. However, the results of the Multisite Multimodal Treatment Study (MTA) shed light on long term outcomes. In this study, outcomes for children with ADHD who had never been medicated were contrasted with those who had been medicated, some of whom were continuing with medications and others who were not. In the long run over eight years, children with ADHD on drugs versus children never on drugs show no difference in results on school achievement. For the MTA study, Molina et al. (2009) noted even those who continued taking medications did not differ from the non-medicated on most measures, with the exception of some benefit for continued drug use on math performance.

Major Depression

The acknowledged fact, even among psychiatrists, is that antidepressants do not work very well even during the eight weeks of initial treatment in adults. Only two-thirds of patients respond to a trial of antidepressant (Thase et al., 2005; Tratner, O'Donovan, Chandarana, and Kennedy, 2002). One half of responders are acknowledged to be placebo responders. Of those who respond to drug, less than half achieve remission from depression (Calabrese et al. 2006; Nemeroff, 2001; Tratner et al. 2002). The previous statements are based on published studies in which the results of treated versus controls did reach statistical significance.

Small reliable differences can be detected when the sample sizes are large enough. On the other hand, in order to be able to recognize when occasionally observed differences are merely chance, and there is in fact no effect, all data must be entered. If some studies which do not show effects are excluded, then there is an increased likelihood that false statistical evidence of effects (particularly small effects) can appear among remaining studies. Irving Kirsch (2010) gathered all the data from antidepressant studies comparing drug to placebo that were reported to the FDA by the drug companies. Analyzing this more complete set of the comparisons between drug and placebo groups, the statistical conclusion was that there was little difference between the groups. The average difference between those treated with an antidepressant versus those receiving placebo is 2 points out of 51 points on the Hamilton Rating Scale, a commonly used assessment measure (Kirsch, Moore, Scoboria, and Nichols, 2002). These results may have contributed to the recent remark by the current director of the National Institute of Mental Health, Thomas Insel (2009), who offered a bottom line on the effectiveness of psychotropic medications in general, when he said: "The unfortunate reality is that current medications help too few people to get better and very few people to get well" (p. 704).

Whereas efficacy of the antidepressants even in the short term is questionable, others have examined the long term outcomes on depression for those taking antidepressants contrasted with outcomes for depression in the pre-drug literature. Giovanni Fava (2003) was an early pioneer in this endeavor. He advanced the hypothesis that current treatments convert an acute problem into a disorder with a chronic course. Fava, and Offidani (2011) reported a similar argument. Littrell (1994) also contrasted outcomes for depression prior to drugs and noted the same pattern of more frequent relapses in those treated with drugs. A recent evaluation by Andrews, Kornstein, Halberstadt, Gardner, and Neale, M. C. (2011) of out comes with antidepressants compared to the depressed but unmedicated reached a similar conclusion. Although the explanations provided for the greater number of relapses over the long run in those taking antidepressants contrasted with those who do not have varied, the worse outcomes in those with drugs has been acknowledged by those who have looked at the data. Littrell (1994) offered drug withdrawal as an explanation for the high rate of depressive symptoms observed in those discontinuing antidepressant medications. Depressive symptoms emerge upon drug discontinuation even in those who were taking antidepressants for anxiety symptoms and who had not been previously depressed (Pato, Zohar-Kadouch, Zohar, and Murphy, 1988).

The efficacy of antidepressant drugs is particularly suspect for children and adolescents. Jureidini et al. (2004) conducted a meta-analysis of the six published randomized controlled studies they could find in the literature evaluating new antidepressants. According to the authors "On 42 reported measures, only 14 showed a statistical advantage for an antidepressant. None of the 10 measures relying on patient reported or parent reported outcomes showed significant advantage for an antidepressant, so that claims for effectiveness were based entirely on ratings by doctors (p. 880)". Two small studies did not find statistical significance. Among the larger studies, two found significant advantage, while two did not. With regard to effect sizes in the positive studies, "the effect size of 0.26 is equivalent to a very modest 3 to 4 point difference on the scale, which has a range of possible scores from 17 to 113 (p. 880)." Thus, the magnitude of the difference between antidepressant treated children's group versus placebo is very small, similar to published results in adults. Consistent with the unclear evidence of efficacy for antidepressants in children, Goodman, Murphy, and Storch (2007) noted that in only 3 of 15 outcome studies submitted to the FDA examining antidepressant efficacy in children for antidepressants were results significant. It should be noted that only fluoxetine/Prozac has been approved by the FDA for treating depression in children, although Prozac, Zoloft/sertraline, and fluvoxamine are approved for treatment of obsessive compulsive disorder.

The largest study of antidepressants in children was the "Treatment of Adolescents with Depression Study" which involved 13 academic centers and 327 adolescents ages 12 to 17 randomly assigned to Cognitive Behavioral Therapy, fluoxetine/Prozac, or a combination. At 12 weeks 73% had experienced a 50% drop in symptoms with combination therapy, compared to 62% with fluoxetine alone, and 48% with CBT. However, by 18 weeks, differences between CBT and fluoxetine were no longer significant. By 24 weeks, differences among treatments were no longer significant on percentages responding to treatment. By 24 weeks, approximately 89% could be counted as responders. In terms of relapses during the 36 months among those who were categorized as responders at 12 weeks, CBT had 3.1% relapses compared to 25.9% relapses in the Prozac group, and 11.5% relapses in the combination group (Rohde et al., 2008). At one year, a point when the researcher did not know what treatments the participants were receiving, a lack of difference among the groups remained. 82.2% of the combined group, 75.2% of the Prozac group, and 70.3% of the CBT group were categorized as responders defined as a 50% drop on scale scores. Recall that responding is not the same as being well. At one year, in terms of those who could be said to be well: 68% of the combined group, 67% of the Prozac, and 69% of the CBT group were described as remitted/well (TADS Team, 2009).

Suicidal events, defined as a suicide attempt, suicidal ideation, or preparatory action toward suicide, but not self-mutilation, were also measured in the TAD study. There were significantly more suicidal events during the 36 weeks with Prozac (14.7%) than with combination (8.4%) or than with CBT (6.3%) (TADS Team, 2007). For newly emergent suicidal events at 12 weeks, the interval during which most of the suicidal events occurred, the numbers were: 11.0% for Prozac; 4.7% for combination; 4.5% for CBT (TADS Team, 2007). Thus, the more rapid response to treatment with Prozac is offset by an increase in the risk for suicidal events.

Dangers of Medications

Anti-Psychotics

Probably the worst side effect of drugs which block the action of dopamine is "brain tissue volume decrement." Ho, Andreasen, Ziebell, Pierson, and Magnotta (2011) tracked first-episode psychotic individuals over an average of seven years. They took brain images over time. They documented a decrease in brain volume that was associated with the dosage of the medication. The effects obtained for both the older (neuroleptics) and the new (atypical) anti-dopaminergic drugs. Ho et al. acknowledged that because they did not observe random assignment to a control group of non-medicated individuals, they could not make a definitive statement that the drugs caused the brain volume decrement. It could have been that those receiving the higher dosages did not come from the same population of individuals. However, Ho et al. cited research with primates. Konopaske et al. (2007; 2008) randomly assigned primates to receive anti-dopaminergic drugs at levels in the therapeutic range for people for 27 months. Those animals who received the drugs exhibited a reduction in total weight of the brain, with greatest reduction in the parietal lobe (with a loss of between 11.8% to 15.2%). Moreover, a 14.2% reduction in glial cell (fat cells) numbers was reported. The glial cell reduction is notable because these cells release growth factors which are vital to maintain the health of the brain (Schwartz and Schechter, 2011; Ziv and Schwartz, 2008). Dopamine, the neurotransmitter blocked by antipsychotic drugs, is a trigger for getting glial cells to release growth factors (Miklic, Juric, Carman-Krzan, 2004). The Konopaske studies are not the only studies in primates. Results similar to Konopaske et al.'s were found in a macaque study by Dorph-Petersen et al. (2005) who noted a 8-11% reduction in brain volume after 1.5 to 2.3 years of exposure to haloperidol (old neuroleptic) or olanzapine (new atypical).

While brain volume reduction may be the most ominous side-effect of the antipsychotic drugs, brain volume reduction is not the only side effect. Atypical antipsychotics are notorious for inducing weight gain that does not plateau, type-2 diabetes, and an increase in fat levels in blood. Children are at elevated risk for developing metabolic side effects (Correll and Carlson, 2006; Safer, 2004; Sikich et al., 2004; Tohen et al., 2007; Woods et al., 2002). The older neuroleptic drugs have long been noted to be associated with Parkinson's symptoms (extra-pyramidal symptoms) in the short term, and permanent movement disorders (tardive dyskinesia) in the long run. The Clinical Antipsychotic Trial of Effectiveness study, a big government funded study, found that newer drugs were also associated with movement disorders, albeit to a lesser extent (Casey, 2006; Manschrek and Boshers, 2007; Miller et al., 2005). The FDA has also issued a warning indicating that the atypicals are associated with QT wave prolongation. Thus, fatal heart arrhythmias can occur (Psychiatric News Alert, 2011).

Lithium

Lithium causes cognitive slowing in adults (Ghaemi, 2008; Pachet and Wisniewski, 2003); impairment is also observed in children (Geller et al., 1998; Silva, 1992). Other annoying side effects include: confusion, slurred speech, ataxia, frequent urination, enuresis, abdominal discomfort, nausea, and vomiting (Hagino et al., 1995). Twenty percent of patients experience weight gain (Chen and Silverstone, 1990). Lithium is associated with thyroid dysfunction (Goodwin and Jamison, 2007). Lithium can cause damage to the cerebellum (Goodwin and Jamison, 2007) and has been associated with cardiac arrhythmias (Ghamei, 2008).

Perhaps most troubling for medicating children is the risk of End Stage Renal Disease in those treated for an extended period of time (over 12 years). In a sample of 74 patients treated for 20 years, 12 reached End Stage Renal Disease (Presne et al., 2003). Presne noted that fifty percent of patients on lithium exhibit impaired renal concentrating ability (Presne et al., 2003). Even when medication is discontinued, kidney damage once started can continue (Markowitz et al., 2000), although kidney damage is related to the duration of lithium treatment (Bendz, Aurell, and Lanke, 2001). Extrapolating from these finding, if children are placed on lithium at age 6, some of them will need a kidney transplant at age 26. People develop an immune response to their transplants even when on immunosuppressants (Galliford and Game, 2009). Approximately, 19% of kidney transplants will be rejected within five years (Murphy, 2010, p. 259). Thus, lithium treatment in children can be expected to significantly shorten life span for some, if not many, of them.

Mood Stabilizers

The annoying side effects of valproate include sedation, nausea, and vomiting. Hematological side effects (anemia, low white counts) have been noted (American Academy of Child and Adolescent Psychiatry, 1997). Up to 89% of young women treated with valproate develop polycystic ovarian disease, involving weight gain, facial hair, and menstrual irregularities (Isojarvi et al., 1993). Valporate increases risk for diabetes (Correll and Carlson, 2006). Both hepatitis and pancreatitis can be induced by valproate and carry black box warnings issued by the FDA (2009). Depression can be induced and both carbamazepine and valproate have black box warnings for suicidal ideations (US FDA, 2008). Anticonvulsants such as valoporate are noted for inducing cognitive impairment (American Academy of Child and Adolescent Psychiatry, 1997; Banu et al., 2007; Loring and Meador, 2004 Henin et al., 2009). Lamotrigene is another mood stabilizer. Lamotrigene is associated with Stevens-Johnson syndrome. Stevens-Johnson's syndrome entails life threatening blistering on all external body surfaces (Borchers, Lee, Naguwa, Cheema, and Gershwin, 2008).

Stimulants

Stimulants include amphetamines and Ritalin/methylphenidate. Adderall is a long acting form of amphetamines, while concerta is a timed-release preparation of Ritalin. Stimulants have a black box warning for heart attacks in Canada and the U.S. (CanWestNews, 2008; Physician's Desk Reference, 2012). Stimulants do suppress growth in height possibly through inhibition of growth hormone (Faraone, Biederman, Morley, Spencer, 2008; Zhang, Du, Zhuang, 2010). Stimulants can induce psychosis and are associated with sleep disturbance and suppression of appetite, and induction of motor tics (Physician's Desk Reference, 2012). Stimulants also suppress playfulness in animals (Beatty, Dodge, Dodge, White, and Panksepp, 1982) . Animal research suggests that the purpose of play in youngsters, which is found cross species, is to facilitate social development and maturation of the orbitofrontal cortex and the Prefrontal Cortex (Bell, Pellis, and Kolb, 2010). Most of the research on stimulants has focused on the impact on concentration and school performance. Very little research has focused on social development. It is however known that stimulants can precipitate mania in the predisposed (DelBello et al., 2001).

As a part of the Individuals with Disabilities Education and Improvement Act of 2004, Schools cannot require children to take a stimulant to stay in school (see AbleChild.org web site).

Anti-Depressants

Selective Serotonin Reuptake Inhibitors carry black box warnings for agitation and suicidal ideation in children and adolescents (US FDA, 2007). Reinblatt, doReis, Walkup, and Riddle (2009) document that the SSRI, fluvoxamine, will induce "activation adverse events" including increased activity, impulsivity, insomnia, and disinhibition, in 45% of children. In adults, loss of libido and sexual dysfunction are common (Rosen, Lane, Menza, 1999). Studies examining the impact of SSRIs on puberty and or later adult sexual functioning are not available, although in adults sexual dysfunction can persist after drug discontinuation (Csoka, Bahrich, Mehtonan, 2008). Studies with adults suggest that taking antidepressants for over a year is associated with weight gain (Fava, 2000; Raeder et al. 2006); an increase in C-Reactive Protein, a risk factor for cardiovascular disease (Hamer et al., 2011); type II diabetes (Kivimäjum et al., 2010; Raeder et al., 2006;Rubin et al., 2010); and metabolic syndrome (Dawood et al., 2007; Kemp et al., 2010); and cognitive impairment (Damsa et al., 2004; Fava, 2006). Brain imaging research investigating the emotional numbing effect of selective serotonin reuptake inhibitors (SSRIs), finds that in persons taking SSRIs emotional response to both positive and negative stimuli are dampened (McCabe, Mishor, Cowen, and Hamer, 2010).

A major problem with initiating treatment with antidepressants is that they are associated with severe withdrawal symptoms when the drug is discontinued. As previously discussed, depression emerges as a component of withdrawal even in those who were taking antidepressants for anxiety and were not initially depressed (Pato, Zohar-Kadouch, Zohar, and Murphy, 1988). Haddad (1997) indicates that 20-86% of sample report symptoms, after discontinuing the drug, which include dizziness, nausea, lethargy, headache, anxiety, tingling and burning sensations, confusion, tremor, sweating, insomnia, irritability, memory problems, anorexia. Stoukides and and Stoukides (1991) provided a case report of man who had taken Prozac/fluoxetine for 6 months, upon discontinuation was experienced muscle spasms and exhibited protruding tongue movements. Consistent with the case report, Ceccherini-Nelli et al. (1993) reported that of 10 individuals examined, seven exhibited withdrawal symptoms which included cardiac arrhythmia, resting tremor of the jaw, tongue, and upper extremities, insomnia, chills, sweating, nausea, headache. Along with other symptoms, Lejoyeux and Adés (1997) reported mania or hypomania, delirium, mood changes, dizziness, sensations of tingling and burning in limbs. Goldstein et al. (1999) and McGrath et al. (1993) also reported the emergence of mania upon withdrawal. Surprisingly, protocols for detoxing patients from antidepressants have not been published. Assuming female foster children will grow up and have normal lives including becoming parents themselves, continuing with SSRIs during pregnancy is problematic. SSRIs increase the risk of autism (Croen, Grether, Yoshida, Odouli, and Hendrick, 2011). Withdrawal symptoms in the infant, heart defects, hypospadias (misplaced urethra opening in the male), and life threatening pulmonary hypertension in the new born have been reported for infants exposed to antidepressants during gestation (Chambers et al., 2006; Gentile, 2011; Udechuku, Nguyen, Hill, and Szego, 2010).

Research on Bipolar I has documented that early onset depression is often a precursor to the emergence of mania (Leverich et al., 2006). Thus, depression in a child is a risk factor for mania. Indeed, Goldberg et al. (2001) found that 19% of their young depressives converted to mania. It is further known that antidepressants can precipitate a mania (Ghaemi, Hsu, Soldani, and Goodwin, 2003). Indeed, antidepressants can precipitate mania in as many as 44% of those who exhibit fluctuations in mood (Akiskal, Djenderedijian, Rosenthal, andKhani, 1977). Thus, the relatively high risk of inducing mania is another danger of using antidepressant medications in young persons.

Forces behind Diagnosing and Medicating Children

At the individual level, some of the incentive for providing strong diagnoses to children derives from the Medicaid system allowing more visits to those children with more extreme diagnoses. Moreover, severe diagnoses may qualify a child for Supplemental Security Income from the Social Security System. Once particular diagnoses are provided, medication seems to follow automatically despite the guidelines of the American Academy of Child and Adolescent Psychiatry (Gleason et al., 2007) that for small children, other interventions should be tried first. The pressures toward diagnosis cannot, however, explain the higher doses of medications exceeding recommendations of the FDA and why so many children received multiple medications. Perhaps one has to look at how doctors are trained and to the financial ties to the pharmaceutical industry of the academic opinion leaders who are running the continuing education programs.

Senator Charles Grassley's committee investigated the ties between academic psychiatrists and the pharmaceutical industry. Both Charles Nemeroff of Emory University and Joseph Biederman of Harvard were sanctioned for failing to reveal the extent of their financial remuneration to their employers (Harris and Carey, 2008a/b). (Biederman, as mentioned previously, was the exponent for the diagnosis of Pediatric Bipolar.) In the Grassely Committee hearings, there was also concern expressed over the ghostwriting of articles and books by the pharmaceutical industry with prominent academicians appending their names to these publications (Grassley, 2010).

Notes of caution against the broad based use of antipsychotics have appeared in the literature. For example, Ho et al. (2011) indicate "our findings may lead to heightened concerns regarding potential brain volume changes associated with the sharp rise in atypical antipsychotic use in non-schizophrenic psychiatric disorders (p. 135)." Dosreis et al. (2011) caution, "Antipsychotic poly-pharmacy has demonstrated greater adverse effects with only marginal benefits" and "Given the lack of scientific evidence for such practice, the lack of data on the cumulative risks on child development, and the clear indications of the metabolic adverse effects with these agents, it is important to investigate concomitant antipsychotic use in this vulnerable child population." Comer, Mojtabai, and Olfson (2011), referring to the rise of atypicals in the treatment of anxiety disorders, indicate "Prudence further suggests that renewed clinical efforts should be made to limit use of these medications to clearly justifiable circumstances (p. 1064)". However, the words of caution provided in the journals may not be enough to drown out advertisements from pharmaceutical houses and the cacophony of opinion leaders tethered to industry.

There is a problem with the system for informing physicians. Doctors do have to accumulate continuing education hours to maintain their licenses. There is no formal mechanism for awarding credit for simply reading journals. Drug companies sponsor and select the speakers for the Continuing Education Programs. All the medical journals are replete with industry advertisements. Given the system for informing doctors, it is no wonder why many physicians, who were writing prescriptions for poly-pharmacy and dosages in excess of those recommended by the FDA, probably believed that they were following good practice.

Alarm and Advocacy

Presently, Allen Frances (2009; 2010a/b), a Co-Chair of the DSM-IV, has led a rebellion against the Committees developing the DSM-V. Frances cautioned against the unintended consequences of the manner in which the DSM-IV criteria were stated, which led to the epidemic rise in the diagnoses for ADHD and Bipolar Disorder (Frances, 2011c).

In an interview with Gary Greenberg (2010), Allen Frances explained his activism, "kids getting unneeded antipsychotics that would make them gain 12 pounds in 12 weeks hit me in the gut. It was uniquely my job and my duty to protect them. If not me to correct it, who? I was stuck without an excuse to convince myself." A petition, entitled "Open letter to the DSM-5", on October 23, 2011, launched by the Society for Humanistic Psychology and several other American Psychological Association divisions, was posted on the Web (http://www.ipetitions.com/petition/dsm5/). The petition implores the DSM-5 committees to avoid further loosening of the criteria for being diagnosed with a mental disorder. Frances (2011a, b) has applauded the effort and has urged others to sign.

A number of physicians have written books detailing how the industry has provided lucrative fees to academic opinion leaders who present the materials carefully prepared by the pharmaceutical industry at continuing "education" conferences. Carl Elliott (2010) in *White Coat, Black Hat* details the lack of ethics in medicine generally and the heavy domination by pharmaceutical houses. Doug Bremner, an Emory psychiatrist who was once an opinion leader on the circuit marketing pharmaceuticals, has a web site where he discusses the side effects of various medications. Doug Bremner (2011), in the *Goose that Laid the Golden Egg* as well as on his website, details his legal entanglements with drug companies when he published a study connecting Accutane, a drug used in the treatment of acne, with increased risk for suicide. Phillip Sinaikin (2010), another individual once on the circuit for the pharmaceuticals, offers witness testimony to corruption of influential members of the psychiatric profession in *Psychiatryland*. Joanna Moncrieff (2003) also detailed the influence of the pharmaceutical industry in *"Is psychiatry for sale?"* Marcia Angell (2005), former editor of the *New England Journal of Medicine*, has written extensively about loss of credibility in the medical profession because of ties to industry. Recently, she (2011) offered a supportive review of Bob Whitaker's (2010) *Anatomy of an Epidemic* in *New York Review of Books*. (Whitaker contrasts outcome pre and post drugs for anitdepressants, mood stabilizers, and antipsychotics and finds that outcomes are worse with drugs.) She concurs that there is a paucity of data on the long term effects of psychotropic medications of any type for any age. Most of the "data" consists of industry funded studies which follow patients for eight weeks.

Others have focused more specifically on the heavy medications being used for foster children. The public broadcasting system program The Watchlist (2011) aired "The Medication of Foster Children". Diane Sawyer ran segments on ABC news documenting the medication of children in foster care during the first week in December of 2011. Jeffery Thompson, a state Medicaid director in Washington state, organized the Medicaid Medical Directors Learning Network (2010) to investigate the practice of medicating foster children with strong medications. Senators Grassley and Landrieu developed the Senate Caucus on Foster Care Youth to investigate the issue of psychotropics (Samuels, 2011). James Gottstein of Psychrights sued the state of Alaska on behalf of foster children. Senator Carper of Delaware held a Committee meeting on December 1, 2011 to hear testimony of experts and to discuss the findings of the GAO on the five state survey on the extent of medicating children in foster care.

Moving Forward

In September of 2011, Congress passed the Child and Family Services Improvement and Innovation Act. This law requires that states applying for certain federal child welfare grants establish protocols for the appropriate use and monitoring of psychotropic drugs prescribed to children. In the GAO's report to congress (Kutz, 2011), they indicated that compliance with the guidelines promulgated by the American Academy of Child and Adolescent Psychiatry requires obtaining informed consent for medical treatment. Unfortunately, the GAO report did not discuss who might be empowered to provide informed consent for foster children. In my personal experience, case workers and foster parents are quite intimidated by doctors and are reluctant to challenge a recommendation. This is consistent with Matt Salo's (2011) testimony before the Carper Sub-Committee indicating that states "had to abandon an attempt to strengthen the hand of foster care workers in these situations, when it became clear that

BA/BS or MSW educated workers would face significant liability issue when disagreeing with prescribers." In fact, foster parents have been accused of medical neglect when they objected to medicating children in their care. Of course, expecting physicians to exercise good judgment has resulted in the extant situation.

On December 1, 2011 Senator Tom Carper of Delaware convened the Senate Sub-Committee on Financial Management, Government Information, Federal Services, and International Security. At this meeting, discussed early in this paper, the GAO announced plans to contact states to develop tracking systems to monitor the medicating of children in foster care. The federal government through National Association of Medical Directors may provide policies on best practice. Jim Gottstein (personal communication, 2011), of Psychrights, also suggests that doctors engaging in off-label prescribing for which there is paucity of justification in the research literature (that is, there is no medically accepted indication), are guilty of Medicaid fraud. Thus, the federal government can act to protect foster children by bringing charges of Medicaid fraud against both doctors and the pharmacies that fill the prescriptions. With regard to children in the general public, on August 1, 2011, Ron Paul has introduced "The Parental Consent Act" (HR2769) which will require informed consent from parents for participation in mental health screening.

Hopefully, more foster children will remain drug free given these new policies. However, assuming that the drugs were at least effective at sedating these children, other supports for foster parents will be needed. This may require more use of behavior therapy and psychotherapy. Evaluation of the cost effectiveness of these interventions should be made. Recently, Fullerton et al. (2011) noted an increase in Medicaid spending for persons with Major Depression which coincided with an increased reliance on atypical antipsychotics. Given the high cost of atypical antipsychotics safer treatment may even be cheaper.

REFERENCES

Able Child Organization (2011). http://www.ablechild.org

Akiskal, H. S., Djenderedjian, A. M., Rosenthal, R. H., and Khani, M. K. (1977). Cyclothymic disorder: validating criteria for inclusion in the bipolar affective group. *American Journal of Psychiatry, 134*(11), 1227-1233.

American Academy of Child and Adolescent Psychiatry. (1997). Practice parameters for the assessment and treatment of children and adolescents with Bipolar Disorder. *Journal of the American Academy of Child and Adolescent Psychiatry, 36* (10 supplement), s157-176.

American Psychiatric Association. (1994). *Diagnostic and Statistical Manual of Mental Disorders, fourth edition.* Washington DC: Author.

American Psychiatric Association. (2000). *Diagnostic and Statistical Manual of Mental Disorders, fourth edition-TR.* Washington DC: Author.

American Psychiatric Association, Mood disorders workgroup. (2011). Issues pertinent to a developmental approach to Bipolar Disorder in DSM-5. 1-6. http://www.dsm5.org

American Psychiatric Association, Childhood and Adolescent Disorders Work Group. (2011). Justification for temper dysregulation disorder with dysphoria. http://www.dsm5.org/proposedrevision.aspx?rid=397.

Amminger, G. P., Schafter, M. R., Papageorgiou, K., Klier, C. M., Cotton, S. M., Harrigan, S. M., Mackinnon, A., McGorry, P. D., and Berger, G. E. (2010). Long-chain ω-3 fatty acids for indicated prevention of psychotic disorders: A randomized, placebo-controlled trial. *Archives of General Psychiatry, 67* (2), 146-154.

Andrews, P. W., Kornstein, S. G., Halberstadt, L. J., Gardner, C. O., and Neale, M. C. (2011). Blue again; perturbational effects of antidepressants suggest monoaminergic homeostasis in major depression. *Frontiers in Psychology, 2,* Article 159, 1-24.

Angell, M. (2005). *The truth about drug companies: how they deceive us and what to do about it.* New York: Random House.

Angell, M. (2011, June 23). Why there is an epidemic of mental illness. *New York Review of Books, LVIII* (11), 20-22.

Angell, M. (2011, July 14). The illusion of psychiatry. *New York Review of Books, LVIII* (12), 20-22.

Angell, M. (2011, August 18). The illusion of psychiatry': An exchange. *New York Review of Books, LVIII* (13), 82-84.

Anthony, J., and Scott, P. (1960). Manic-depressive psychosis in childhood. *Journal of Child Psychology and Psychiatry, 4,* 53-72.

Baethge, C., Tondo, L., Bratti, I. M., Bschor, T., Bauer, M., Viguera, A. C., and Baldessarini, R. J. (2003). Prophylaxis latency and outcome in bipolar disorders. *Canadian Journal of Psychiatry, 48* (7), 449-457.

Baldessarini, R. J., Tondo, L., Baethge, C. L., and Bratti, I. M. (2007). Effect of treatment latency on response to maintenance treatment in manic-depressive disorders. *Bipolar Disorder, 9,* 386-393.

Banu, S. H., Jahan, M., Koli, U. K., Ferdousi, S., Khan, N. Z., and Neville, B. (2007). Side effects of Phenobarbital and carbamazepine in childhood epilepsy: randomized controlled trial. *British Medical Journal, 334,* 1207-1213.

Beatty, W.W., Dodge, A. M., Dodge, L. J., White, K., and Panksepp, J. (1982). Psychomotor stimulants, social deprivation, and play in juvenile rats. *Pharmacology, Biochemistry, and Behavior, 16*(3), 417-422.

Bell, H.C., Pellis, S. M., Kolb, B. (2010). Juvenile peer play experience and the development of the orbitofrontal and medial prefrontal cortices. *Behavior and Brain Research, 207*(1), 7-13.

Bendz, H., Aurell, M., and Lanke, J. (2001). A historical cohort study of kidney damage in long-term lithium patients: continued surveillance needed. *European Psychiatry, 16,* 199-206.

Biederman, J., Faraone, S., Mick, E., Wozniak, J., Chen, L., Ouellette, C., Marrs, A., Moore, P., Garcia, J., Mennin, D., and Lelon, E. (1996). Attention-deficit hyperactivity disorder and juvenile mania: A overlooked co-morbidity? *Journal of the American Academy of Child and Adolescent Psychiatry, 35,* 997-1008.

Biederman, J., Klein, K. R., Pine, D.S., and Klein, D. F. (1998). Resolved: mania is mistaken for ADHD in prepubertal children. *Journal of the American Academy of Child and Adolescent Psychiatry, 37* (10), 1091-1096.

Blader, J. C., and Carlson, G. A. (2007). Increased rates of bipolar disorder diagnoses among U.S. child, adolescent, and adult inpatients, 1996-2004. *Biological Psychiatry, 62* (2), 107-114.

Borchers, A. T., Lee, J. L., Naguwa, S. M., Cheema, G. S., and Gershwin, M. E. (2008). Stevens-Johnson syndrome and toxic epidermal necrolysis. *Autoimmune Review, 7* (8), 598-605.

Breland-Noble, A.M., Elbogen, E. B., Farmer, E. M.Z., Wagner, H. R., and Burns, B. J. (2004). Use of psychotropic medications for youths in therapeutic foster care and group homes. *Psychiatric Services, 55* (6), 706-708.

Bremner, J. D. (2011). *The goose that laid the golden egg: Accutane—the truth that had to be told.* UK: Nothing but Publishing Ltd.

Burns, B. J., Phillips, S. D., Wagner, H. R., Barth, R., Kolko, D. J., Campbell, Y., and Landsverk, J. (2004). Mental health need and access to mental health services by youths involved with child welfare: A national study. *Journal of the American Academy of Child and Adolescent Psychology, 43*, 960-970.

Calabreses, J. R., Muzina, D. J., Kemp, D.E., Sachs, G. S., Frye, M. A., Thompson, T.R., Klingman, D., Reed, M. L., Hirschfeld, R. M. A., Harris, T. H., and Davis, H. K. (2006). Predictors of Bipolar Disorder risk among patients currently treated for major depression. *MedGenMed 8* (3), 38.

CanWestNewsService (2006, May 27). Deadly side-effects earn ADHD drugs warning. http:www.canada.com/topics/news/national/story.html?id=375b4d0d-75c4-4b1d-880c-560ce953a8cb

Casey, D. E. (2006). Implications of the CATIE trial on treatment: extrapyramidal symptoms. *CNS Spectrum, 11* (Suppl. 7), 25-31.

Ceccherini-Nelli, A., Bardelllini, L., Cur, A., Guazzelli, M., Maggini, C., and Dilsaver, S. C. (1993). Anti-depressant withdrawal: prospective findings. *American Journal of Psychiatry, 150*, 165.

Chambers, C. D., Hernandez-Diaz, S., Van Marter, L.J., Werier, M. M., Louik, C., Jones, K.L., Mitchell, A. A. (2006). Selective serotonin-reuptake inhibitors and risk of persistent pulmonary hypertension of the newborn. *New England Journal of Medicine, 354*(6), 579-587.

Chang, K. D. (2010). Course and impact of bipolar disorder in young patients. *Journal of Clinical Psychiatry, 71* (2), doi:10.488/JCP.8125tx7c

Chang, K., Howe, M., Gallelli, K., and Miklowitz, D. (2006). Prevention of pediatric bipolar disorder: Integration of neurobiological and psychosocial processes. *Annals of the New York Academy of Sciences, 1094*, 235-247.

Chang, K., and Kowatch, R. A. (2007). Is this child bipolar? What's needed to improve diagnosis? *Current Psychiatry, 6* (10) 23-33.

Chen, Y., and Silverstone, T. (1990). Lithium and weight gain. *International Clinical Psychopharmacology, 5*(3), 217-225.

Child and Family Services Improvement and Innovation Act, September 2011Public L. No. 112-34, § 101(b)(2), 125 Stat. 369.

Comer, J. S., Mojtabai, R., and Olfson, M. (2011). National trends in the antipsychotic treatment of psychiatric outpatients with anxiety Disorders. *American Journal of Psychiatry 168* (10), 1057-1065.

Correll, C. U., and Carlson, H. E. (2006). Endocrine and metabolic adverse effects of psychotropic medications in children and adolescents. *Journal of the American Academy of Child and Adolescent Psychiatry, 45*, 771-791.

Coryell, W., Coryell, J., Endicott, T., Reich, N., Andreasen, N., and Keller, M. (1984). A family study of bipolar II disorder. *British Journal of Psychiatry, 145*, 49-54.

Coryell, W., Endicott, J., Maser, J. D., Keller, M. B., Leon, A. C., and Akiskal, H. S. (1995). Long-term stability of polarity distinctions in the affective disorders. *American Journal of Psychiatry, 152* (3), 385-390.

Croen, L. A., Grether, J.K., Yoshida, C. K., Odouli, R., and Hendrick, V. (2011). Antidepressant use during pregnancy and childhood autism spectrum disorders. *Archives of General Psychiatry, 68* (11), 1104-1112.

Crystal, S., Olfson, M., Huang, C., Pincus, H., and Gerhard, T. (2009). Broadened use of atypical antipsychotics: safety, effectiveness, and policy challenges. *Health Affairs (Millwood), 28*(5), w770-781.

Csoka, A. B., Bahrick, A., Mehtonen, O. P. (2008). Persistent sexual dysfunction after discontinuation of selective serotonin reuptake inhibitors. *Journal of Sexual Medicine, 5* (1), 227-233.

Damsa, C., Bumb, A., Bianchi-Demicheli, F., Vidailhet, P., Sterck, R., Andreoli, A., and Beyenburg, S. (2004). "Dopamine-dependent" side effects of selective serotonin reuptake inhibitors: a clinical review. *Journal of Clinical Psychiatry, 65* (8), 1064-1068.

Dawood, T., Lambert, E. A., Barton, D. A., Laude, D., Elghozi, J. L., Esler, M. D., Haikerwal, D., Kaye, D. M., Hotchkin, E. J., and Lambert, G. W. (2007). Specific serotonin reuptake inhibitors in major depressive disorder adversely affects novel cardiac risk. *Hypertension Research, 30*, 285-293.

DelBello, M. P., Soutullo, C. A., Hendricks, W., Niemeier, R. T., McElroy, S. L., and Strakowski, S. M. (2001). Prior stimulant treatment in adolescents with bipolar disorder: Association with age of onset. *Bipolar Disorders, 2*, 53-57.

Dickstein, D. P., Towbin, K. E., Van Der Veen, J. W., Rich, B. A., Brotman, M. A., Knopf, L., Onello, L., Pine, D. S., Leibenfult, E. (2009). Randomized double-blind placebo-controlled trial of lithium in youth with severe mood dysregulation. *Journal of Child and Adolescent Psychopharmacology, 19*, 61-73.

Domino, M. E., and Swartz, M. S. (2008). Who are the new users of antipsychotic medications? *Psychiatric Services, 59* (5), 507-514.

Dorph-Petersen, K-A., Pierri, J. N., Perel, J. M., Sun, Z., Sampson, A. R., and Lewis, D. A. (2005). The influence of chronic exposure to antispsychotic medications on brain size before and after tissue fixation: a comparison of haldoperiodol and olanzapine in macaque monkeys. *Neuropsychopharmacology, 30*, 1649-1661.

dosReis, S., Zito, J. M., Safer, D.J., and Soken, K. L. (2001). Mental health services for youths in foster care and disabled youths. *American Journal of Public Health, 91*, 1094-1099.

dosReis, S., Yoon, Y., Rubin, D. M., Riddle, M. A., Noll, E., and Rothbard, A. (2011). Antipsychotic treatment among youth in foster care. *Pediatrics*, 128 (6), 1459-1466.

Duffy, A., Alda, M., Hajek, T., and Grof, P. (2009). Early course of bipolar disorder in high-risk offspring: Prospective study. *British Journal of Psychiatry, 195*, 457-458.

Elliot, C. (2010). *White coat, black hat: adventures on the dark side of medicine*. Boston: Beacon Press.

Faraone, S. V., Biederman, J., Morley, C. P., and Spencer, T. J. (2008). Effect of stimulants on height and weight: a review of the literature. *Journal of the American Academy of Child and Adolescent Psychiatry, 47* (9), 994-1009.

Fava, G. A. (2003). Can long-term treatment with antidepressant drugs worsen the course of depression? *Journal of Clinical Psychiatry, 64*(2), 123-133.

Fava, G. A., and Offidani, E. (2011). The mechanisms of tolerance in antidepressant action. *Progress in Neuropsychopharmacology and Biological Psychiatry*, 35 (7), 1593-1602.

Fava, M. (2000). Weight gain and antidepressants. *Journal of Clinical Psychiatry, 61* (Supplement 11), 37-41.

Fava, M. (2006). A cross-sectional study of the prevalence of cognitive and physical symptoms during long-term antidepressant treatment. *Journal of Clinical Psychiatry, 67*, 1754-1759.

Frances, A. (2009, June 26). A warning sign on the road to the DSM-V: beware of its unintended consequences. *Psychiatric Times, 26* (8).

Frances, A. (2010a, March 1). It's not too late to save 'normal'. *Los Angeles Times.* http://articles.latimes.com/2010/mar/01/opinion/la-oe-frances1-201mar01.

Frances, A. (2010b, July 6). Normality is an endangered species: Psychiatric fads and overdiagnosis. *Psychiatric Times.* http://www.psychiatrictimes.com/display/article/10168/1598676

Frances, A. (2011a, November 11). DSM-5: living document or dead on arrival? *Psychiatric Times.* http://www.psychiatrictimes.com/blog/dsm-5/content/article/10168/1989691

Frances, A. (2011b, November 10) The user's revolt against DSM-5: will it work? *Psychiatric Times.* http://www.psychiatrictimes.com/blog/dsm-5/content/article/10168/1988483

Frances, A. (2011c, November 5). Allen Frances: why psychiatrists should sign the petition to reform DSM 5: the fight for the future of psychiatry. http:societyforhumanistic psyhchology.blogspot.com/2011/11/allen-frances-why-psychiatrists-should-sign-the-petition.

Fullerton, C. A., Busch, A. B., Normand, S-T. T., McGuire, T. G., and Epstein, A. M. (2011). Ten-year trends in quality of care and spending for depression: 1996 through 2005. *Archives of General Psychiatry, 66* (12), 1218-1226.

Galliford, J., and Game, D. S. (2009). Modern renal transplantation: present challenges and future prospects. *Postgraduate Medical Journal, 85*, 91-101.

Geller, B., Cooper, T. B., Zimerman, B., Frazier, J., Williams, M., Heath, J., and Warner, K. (1998). Lithium for prepubertal depressed children with family history predictors of future bipolarity: a double-blind, placebo-controlled study. *Journal of Affective Disorders, 51*, 165-175.

Gentile, S. (2011). Drug treatment for mood disorders in pregnancy. *Current Opinion in Psychiatry, 24*(1), 34-40.

Ghaemi, S. N. (2008). *Practical guides in psychiatry: mood disorders, 2nd ed.* New York: Lippincott, Williams, and Wilkins.

Ghaemi, S. N., Hsu, D. J., Soldani, F., and Goodwin, F. K. (2003). Antidepressants in bipolar disorder: The case for caution. *Bipolar Disorders, 5*, 421-433.

Gleason, M. M., Egger, H.L., Emslie, G. J., Greenhill, L. L., Kowatch, R. A., Lieberman, A. F., Luby, J.L., Owens, J., Schahill, L. D., Scheeringa, M. S., Stafford, B., Wise, B., and Zeanah, C.H. (2007). Pharmacological treatment for very young children: Context and guidelines. *Journal of the American Academy of Child and Adolescent Psychiatry, 46*, 1532-1572.

Goldberg, J. F., Harrow, M., and Whiteside, J. E. (2001). Risk for bipolar illness in patients initially hospitalized for unipolar depression. *American Journal of Psychiatry, 15,* 1265-1270.

Goldstein, T. R., Frye, M. A., Denicoff, K. D., Smith-Jackson, E., Leverich, G. S., Bryan, A. L., Ali, S. O. and Post, R. M. (1999). Antidepressant discontinuation-related mania: critical prospective observation and theoretical implications in bipolar disorder. *Journal of Clinical Psychiatry, 60,* 563-567.

Goodman, W. K., Murphy, T. K., and Storch, E. A. (2007). Risk of adverse behavioral effects with pediatric use of antidepressants. *Psychopharmacology, 191,* 87-96.

Goodwin F. K., and Jamison, K. R. (2007). *Manic-depressive illness: bipolar disorders and recurrent depression, 2nd ed.* New York: Oxford Press.

Grassley, C.E. (2010, June 24). Ghostwriting in Medical Literature, Minority Staff Report, 111th Congress; U.S. Senate Committee on Finance. http://www.grassley.senate.gov/ about/upload/Senator-Grassley-Report.pdf

Greenberg, G. (2010, December 10). Inside the battle to define mental illness [Web log post]. Retrieved from www.wired.com /magazine/2010/12/ff_dsmv/all/1 on 3/1/11

Haddad, P. (1997). New antidepressants and the discontinuation syndrome. *Journal of Clinical Psychiatry, 58,* Supplement 7, 17-21.

Hagino, O. R., Weller, E. B., Weller, R. A., Washing, D., Fristad, M. A., Kontras, S. B. (1995). Untoward effects of lithium treatment in children aged four through six years. *Journal of the American Academy of Child and Adolescent Psychiatry, 34,* 1584-1590.

Hamer, M., Batty, G. D., Marmot, M. G., Singh-Manoux, A., and Kivimäki, M. (2011). Antidepressant medication use and C-reactive protein: results from two population-based studies. *Brain, Behavior, and Immunity, 25,* 168-173.

Harris, G., and Carey, B. (2008a, June 8). Researchers fail to reveal full drug pay: Possible conflicts seen in Child Psychiatry, *New York Times.* Retried October 3, 2008 from http://www.nytimes.com

Harris, G., and Carey, B. (2008b, July 12). Psychiatric Association faces Senate scrutiny over drug industry ties. *New York Times,* A 13.

Harrow, M., Goldberg, J. F., Grossman, L. S., and Meltzer, H. Y. (1990). Outcome in manic disorders. *Archives of General Psychiatry, 47* (7), 665-671.

Hart, C. L., Ksir, C., and Ray, O. (2009). *Drugs, society, and human behavior, 13th edition.* New York: McGraw Hill.

Henin, A., Mick, E., Biederman, J., Fried, R., Hirshfeld-Becker, D. R., Micco, J. A., Miller, K. G., Rycyna, C.C., and Wozniak, J. (2009). Is psychopharmacologic treatment associated with neuropsychological deficits in bipolar youth? *Journal of Clinical Psychiatry, 70* (8), 1178-1185.

Ho, B-C., Andreasen, N. C., Ziebell, S., Pierson,m R., and Magnotta, V. (2011). Long-term antipsychotic treatment and brain volume. *Archives of General Psychiatry, 68* (2), 128-137.

Insel, T. R. (2009). Disruptive insights in psychiatry: transforming a clinical discipline. *Journal of Clinical Investigation. 119* (4), 700-705.

Isojarvi, JIT, Laatikainen, T. J., Pakarienen, A. J., Juntunen K.T.S., Myllyla, V. V. (1993). Polycystic ovaries and hyperandrogenism in women taking valporate for epilepsy. *New England Journal of Medicine, 329,* 1383-1388.

Judd, L. L., Akiskal, H. S., Schettler, P. J., Coryell, W., Maser, J., Rice, J. A., Solomon, D. A., and Keller, M. B. (2003). The comparative clinical phenotype and long term longitudinal episode course of bipolar I and II: a prospective, comparative, longitudinal study. *Journal of Affective Disorders, 73*, 19-32.

Judd, L. L., Akiskal, H. S., Schettler, P. J., Endicott, J., Maser, J., Solomon, D. A., Leon, A. C., Rice, J. A., and Keller, M. B. (2002). The long-term natural history of the weekly symptomatic status of Bipolar I Disorder. *Archives of General Psychiatry, 59*, 530-537.

Jureidini, J. JN., Doecke, C. J., Mansfield, P. R., Haby, M. M., Menkes, D. B., and Tonkin, A. L. (2004). Efficacy and safety of antidepressants for children and adolescents. *British Medical Journal, 328*, 879-883.

Kemp, A. H., Quintana, D. S., Gray, M. A., Felmingham, K. L., Brown, K., and Gatt, J. (2010). Impact of depression and antidepressant treatment on heart rate variability: a review and meta-analysis. *Biological Psychiatry, 67*, 1067-1074.

Kiecolt-Glaser, J. K. (2010). Stress, food, and inflammation: psychoneuroimmunology and nutrition at the cutting edge. *Psychosomatic Medicine, 72*(4), 365-369.

Kiecolt-Glaser, J. K., Belury, M. A., Andridge, R., Malarkey, W. B., and Glaser, R. (2011). Omega-3 supplementation lowers inflammation and anxiety in medical students: a randomized controlled trial. *Brain, Behavior,and Immunity, 25*(8), 1725-1734.

Kirsch, I. (2010). *The emperor's new drugs: exploding the antidepressant myth*. New York: Basic Books.

Kirsch, I., Moore, T. J., Scoboria, A., and Nicholls, S. S. (2002). The emperor's new drugs: an analysis of antidepressant medication data submitted to the U.S. Food and Drug Administration. *Prevention and Treatment*, Vol5, Article 2, Copyright by American Psychological Association.

Kivimäjum N., Hamer, M., Batty, G. D., Geddes, J. R., Tabak, A. G., Pentti, J., Virtanen, M., and Vahtera, J. (2010). Antidepressant medication use, weight gain, and risk of Type 2 diabetes. *Diabetes Care, 33* (12), 2611-2616.

Konopaske, G. T., Dorph-Petersen, K-A., Pierri, J. N., Wu, Q., Sampson, A. R., and Lewis, D. A. (2007). Effect of chronic exposure to antipsychotic medication on cell numbers in the parietal cortex of the macaque monkeys. *Neuropsychopharmacology, 32*, 1216-1223.

Konopaske, G. T., Dorph-Petersen, K-A., Sweet, R. A., Pierri, J. N., Zhang, W., Sampson, A. R., and Lewis, D. A. (2008). Effect of chronic antipsychotic exposure on astrocyte and oligodendrocyte numbers in macaque monkeys. *Biological Psychiatry, 63*, 759-765.

Kutz, G. D. (2011) United States Accountability Office Testimony before the Subcommittee on Federal Financial Management, Government Information, Federal Services, and International Security, Committee on Homeland Security and Governmental Affairs, U.S. Senate. December 1, 2011; Gregory D. Kutz, Director Forensic Audits and Investigative Service

Lejoyeux, M., and Adés, J. (1997). Antidepressant discontinuation: a review of the literature. *Journal of Clinical Psychiatry, 58* (Supplement 7), 11-15.

Leslie, L., Kelleher, K., Burns, B., Landsverk, J., and Rolls, J. (2003). Foster care and Medicaid managed care. *Child Welfare League of America, 82*(3), 367-392.

Leverich, G. S., Alshuler, L. L., Frye, M. A., Suppes, T., McElory, S. L., Keck, P. E., Kupka, R. W., Denicoff, K. D., Nolen, W. A., Grunze, H., Martinez, M. I., and Post, R. M. (2006). Risk of switch in mood polarity to hypomania or mania in patients with bipolar depression during acute and continuation trials of venlafaxine, sertraline, and bupropion as adjuncts to mood stabilizers. *American Journal of Psychiatry, 163,* 232-239.

Littrell, J. (1994). Relationship between time since reuptake-blocker antidepressant discontinuation and relapse. *Experimental and Clinical Psychopharmacology, 2* (1), 82-94.

Littrell, J. and Lyons, P. (2010a). Pediatric Bipolar Disorder: Part I—Is it related to classical Bipolar? *Children and Youth Services Review, 32*(7), 945-964.

Littrell, J., and Lyons, P. (2010b) . Pediatric Bipolar Disorder: An issue for child welfare. *Children and Youth Services Review, 32*(7), 965-973.

Loranger, A., and Levine, P. (1978). Age at onset of bipolar affective illness. *Archives of General Psychiatry, 35,* 1345-1348.

Loring, D. W., and Meador, K. J. (2004). Cognitive side effects of antiepileptic drugs in children. *Neurology, 62,* 872-877.

Manschreck, T. C., and Boshes, R. A. (2007). The CATIE schizophrenia trail: results, impact, and controversy. *Harvard Review of Psychiatry, 15*(5), 245-258.

Markowitz, G. S., Radhakrishnan, J., Kambham, N., Valeri, A. M., Hines, W. H., and D'Agatti, V.D. (2000). Lithium nephrotoxicity: A progressive combined glomerular and tubulointerstitial nephropathy. *Journal of the American Society of Nephrology, 11,* 1439-1448.

Marshall, M., Lewis, S., Lockwood, A., Drake, R., Jones, P., and Croudace, T., (2005). Association between duration of untreated psychosis and outcome in cohorts of first-episode patients: a systematic review. *Archives of General Psychiatry, 62* (9), 975-983.

Marshall, M., and Rathbone, J. (2011a). Early intervention for psychosis. *The Cochrane Data Base Systematic Reviews, 6,* CD004187

Marshall, M., and Rathbone, J. (2011b). Early intervention for psychosis. *Schizophrenia Bulletin, 37* (6), 1111-1114.

Martin, A., Young, C., Leckman, J. P., Mukonoweschuro, C., Rosenheck, R., and Leslie, D. (2004). Age effects in antidepressant-induced manic conversion. *Archives of Pediatric Adolescent Medicine, 158*(8), 773-780.

Medicaid Medical Directors Learning Network and Rutgers Center for Education and Research on Mental Health Therapeutics. (2010, July) Antipsychotic Medication Use in Medicaid Children and Adolescents: Report and Resource Guide from a 16-state study, MMDLN/Rutgers CERTs, Publication 1 http://rci.rutgers.edu/~cseap/MMDL NAPKIDS/Antipsychotic_Use_in_Medicaid_Children_Report_and_Resource_Guide_F inal.pdf

McCabe, C.,Mishor, Z., Cowen, P. J., and Harmer, C. J. (2010). Diminished neural processing of aversive and rewarding stimuli during selective serotonin reuptake inhibitor treatment. *Biological Psychiatry, 67* (5), 439-445.

McGrath, P. J., Stewart, J. W., Tricamo, E., Nunes, E. N., and Quitkin, F. M. (1993). Paradoxical mood shifts to euthytmia or hypomania upon withdrawal of antidepressant agents. *Journal of Clinical Psychopharmacology, 13*(3), 224-225.

Miklic, S., Juric, D. M., and Carman-Krzan, M. (2004). Differences in the regulation of bdnf and ngf synthesis in cultured neonatal rat astrocytes. *International Journal of Developmental Neuroscience, 22,* 119-130.

Molina, B.S.G., Hinshaw, S.P., Swanson, J. M., Arnold, L.E., Vitiello, B., Jensen, P. S., Epstein, J. N., Hoza, B., Hechtman, L., Abikoff, H. W., Elliot, G. R., Greenhill, L. L.,

Newcorn, J.H., Well, K. C., Wigal, T., Gibbons, R. D., Hur, K., Houck, P.S. and MTA Cooperative Group. (2009). The MTA at 8 years: Prospective follow-up of children treated for combined type ADHD in a Multisite Study. *Journal of the American Academy of Child and Adolescent Psychiatry, 48*(5), 484-500.

Miller, D. D., EcVoy, J.P. Davis, S. M.< Caroff, S. N., Saltz, B. L., Chakos, M. H., Swartz, M. S., Keefe, R. S., Rosenheck, R. A., Stroup, T. S., and Lieberman, J. A. (2005). Clinical correlates of tardive dyskinesia in schizophrenia: baseline data from the CATIE schizophrenia trail. *Schizophrenia Research, 80*(1), 33-43.

Moncrieff, J. (2003). Is psychiatry for sale? Maudsley discussion paper. Available as booklet from the institute of psychiatry sarah.smith@iop.kcl.ac.uk.

Moreno, C., Laje, G., Blanco, C., Jiang, H., Schmidt, A. B., and Olfson, M. (2007). National trends in the outpatient diagnosis and treatment of bipolar disorder in youth. *Archives of General Psychiatry, 64* (9), 1032-1039.

Murphy, K. (2012). *Janeway's Immunobiology.* New York: Garland Science.

Nemeroff, C. B. (2001). Progress in the battle with the black dog: Advances in the treatment of depression. *American Journal of Psychiatry, 158* (10), 1555-1557.

Pachet, A. K., and Wisniewski, A. M. (2003). The effects of lithium on cognition: an updated review. *Psychopharmacology, 170,* 225-234.

Pato, M. T., Zohar-Kadouch, R., Zohar, J., and Murphy, D. L. (1988). Return of symptoms after discontinuation of clomipramine in patients with obsessive-compulsive disorder. *American Journal of Psychiatry, 145,* 1521-1525.

Perkins, D. D., Gu, H., Boteva, K., Lieberman, J. A. (2005). Relationship between duration of untreated psychosis and outcome in first-episode schizophrenia: a critical review and meta-analysis. *American Journal of Psychiatry, 162* (10), 1785-1804.

Physicians' desk reference, (66 edition). (2012). Montvale, NJ: PDR Network.

Post, R. (2004). Neurobiology of seizures and behavioral abnormalities. *Epilepsia, 45,* (Suppl. 2), 5-14.

Post, R. M. (2007). Kindling and sensitization as models for affective episode recurrence, cyclicity, and tolerance phenomena. *Neuroscience and Biobehavioral Reviews, 31,* 858-873.

Post, R. M., Denicoff, K. D., Leverich, G. S., Altschuler, L. L., Frye, M. A., Suppes, T. M., Rush, A. J., Keck, P. E., McElroy, S. L., Luckenbaugh, D. A., Pollio, C., Kupka, R., and Nolen, W. A. (2003). Morbidity in 258 bipolar outpatients followed for 1 year with daily prospective ratings on the NIMH life chart method. *Journal of Clinical Psychiatry, 64* (6), 680-690.

Postma, T., Krupp, E., Li, X. L., Post, R. M., and Weiss, S.R. (2000). Lamotrigine treatment during amygdala-kindled seizure development fails to inhibit seizures and diminishes subsequent anticonvulsant efficacy. *Epilepsia, 41*(12), 1514-1521.

Presne, C., Fakhouri, F., Noël, L-H., Stengel, B., Even, C., Kreis, H., Mignon, F., and Grönfeld, J-P. (2003). Lithium-induced nephropathy: Rate of progression and prognostic factors. *Kidney International, 64,* 585-592.

Psychiatric News Alert (2011, July 21). *FDA orders new warning on Seroquel label.* http://alert.psychiatricnews.org/2011/03/fda-order-new-warning-on-seroquel.html.

Psychrights (2011). http:psychrights.org/index.htm.

Raeder, M. B., Bjelland, I., Emil Vollset, S., and Steen, V. M. (2006). Obesity, dyslipidemia, and diabetes with selective serotonin reuptake inhibitors: the Hordaland Health Study. *Journal of Clinical Psychiatry, 67* (2), 1947-1982.

Raghavan, R., and McMillen, J. C. (2007). Patterns of psychotropic medication use among older adolescents in foster care. *Academy Health Annual Research Meeting*. Orlando, FL.

Raghavan, R., Zima, B. T., Andersen, R. M., Leibowitz, A. A., Schuster, M. A., and Landsverk, J. (2005). Psychotropic medication use in a National Probability sample of children in the child welfare system. *Journal of Child and Adolescent Psychopharmacology, 15,* 97-106.

Reinblatt, S. P., dosReis, S., Walkup, J. T., and Riddle, M. A. (2009). Activation adverse events induced by selective serotonin reuptake inhibitor fluvoxamine in children and adolescents. *Journal of Child and Adolescent Psychopharmacology, 19*(2), 119-136.

Rennie, T. A. C. (1942). Prognosis in manic-depressive psychosis. *American Journal of Psychiatry, 98,* 801-814.

Rohde, P., Silva, S. G., Tonev, S. T., Kennard, B. D., Vitiello, B., Kratochvil, C. J., Reinecke, M. A., Curry, J. F., Simons, A. D., and March, J. S. (2008). Achievement and maintenance of sustained response during the TADS continuation and maintenance therapy. *Archives of General Psychiatry, 65*(4), 447-455.

Rosen, R. C., Lane, R. M., and Menza, M. (1999). Effects of SSRIs on sexual function: a critical review. *Journal of Clinical Psychopharmacology, 19* (1), 67-85.

Rubin, R. R., Ma, Y., Peyrot, M., Marrero, D. G., Price, D.W., Barrett-Connor, E., Knowler, W. C. (2010). Antidepressant medicine use and risk of developing diabetes during the diabetes prevention program and diabetes prevention program outcome study. *Diabetes Care, 33* (12), 2549-2551.

Safer, D. J. (2004). A comparison of risperidone-induced weight gain across the life span. *Journal of Clinical Psychopharmacology, 24,* 429-436.

Salo, M. (2011, December 1). The financial and societal cost of medicating America's foster children. Testimony of Executive Director for the National Association of Medicaid Directors before the Senate Homeland Security and Government Affairs Committee. http://hsgac.senate.gov/public/index.cfm?FuseAction=Hearings.HearingandHearing_Ib=9fc1 94de-2a7c-4417-8f2b-6b90cadacede

Samuels, B. (2011, December 1). Testimony of the Commissioner form Administration of Children, Youth and Families and Administration of Children and Families, U.S. Department of Health and Human Services before the Senate Homeland Security and Government Affairs Committee. http://hsgac.senate.gov/public/index.cfm?FuseAction= Hearings.HearingandHearing_Ib=9fc194de-2a7c-4417-8f2b-6b90cadacede

Schwartz, M., and Schechter, R. (2011). Systemic inflammatory cells fight off neurodegenerative disease. *Nature Reviews: Neurology, 6,* 405-410.

Sikich, L., Hamer, R. M., Bashford, R. A., Sheitman, B. B., and Lieberman, J. A. (2004). A pilot study of risperidone, olanzapine and haloperidol in psychotic youth: A double-blind, randomized, 8-week trial. *Neuropsychopharmacology, 29,* 133-145.

Silva, R. R., Campbell, M., Golden, R. R., Small, A. M., Pataki, C. S., and Rosenberg, C. R. (1992). Side effects associated with lithium and placebo administration in aggressive children. *Psychopharmacology Bulletin, 28* (3), 319-326.

Sinaikin, P. (2010). *Psychiatryland*. New York: iUniverse, Inc.

Soetens, E., E'Hooge, R., and Hueting, J.E. (1993). Amphetamine enhances human-memory consolidation. *Neuroscience Letter, 161* (1), 9-12.

Sostek, A. J., Buchsbaum, M. S., and Rapoport, J. L. (1980). Effects of amphetamine on vigilance performance in normal and hyperactive children. *Journal of Abnormal Child Psychology, 8*(4), 491-500.

Spetie, L., and Arnold, L. E. (2007). Ethical issues in child psychopharmacology research and practice: Emphasis on preschoolers. *Psychopharmacology, 191,* 15-26.

Stahmer, A. C., Leslie, L. K., Hurlburt, M. S., Barth, R., Webb, M. B., Landsverk, J.A. and Zhang, J. (2005). Developmental and behavioral needs and service use for young children in child welfare. *Pediatrics, 116,* 891-900.

Stoukides, J.A., and Stoukides, C. A. (1991). Extrapyramidal symptoms upon discontinuation of fluoxetine. *American Journal of Psychiatry, 148,* 1263.

Thase, M. E., Haight, B. R., Richard, N., Rockett, C. B., Mitton, M., Modell, J. G., VanMeter, S., Harriett, A.E., and Wang, Y. (2005). Remission rates following antidepressant therapy with bupropion or selective serotonin reuptake inhibitors: a meta-analysis of original data from 7 randomized controlled trials. *Journal of Clinical Psychiatry, 66* (8), 974-981.

Thompson, A., Nelson, B., and Yung, A. (2011). Predictive validity of clinical variables in the "at risk" for psychosis population: international comparison with results from the North American Prodrome Longitudinal Study. *Schizophrenia Research, 126* (1-3), 51-57.

Tohen, M., Kryzhanovskaya, L, Carlson, G., DelBello, M., Wozniak, J., Kowatch, R., Wagner, K., Findling, R., Lin, D., Robertson-Plouch, C., Xu, W., Dittmann, R. W., and Biederman, J. (2007). Olanzapine versus placebo in the treatment of adolescents with bipolar mania. *American Journal of Psychiatry, 164,* 1547-1556.

Tranter, R., O'Donovan, C., Chandarana, P., and Kennedy, S. (2002). Prevalence and outcome of partial remission in depression. *Journal of Psychiatry and Neuroscience, 27* (4), 241-247.

TADS (2007). The Treatment for Adolescents with Depression Study. *Archives of General Psychiatry, 64*(10), 1132-1144.

TADS (2009). The Treatment for Adolescents with Depression Study(TADS): outcomes over 1 year naturalistic follow-up. *American Journal of Psychiatry, 166,* 1141-1149

Tyre, P. (2004, December). Battling the effects of war. Newsweek. Retrieved September 14, 2008. from http://www.newsweek.com/id/5598

Udachina, A., and Mansell, W. (2007). Cross-validation of the mood disorders questionnaire, the internal state, and the hypomanic personality scale. *Personality and Individual Differences, 42,* 1539-1549.

Udechucku, A., Nguyen, T., Hill, R, and Szego, K. (2010). Antidepressants in pregnancy: a systemic review. *Australian and New Zealand Journal of Psychiatry, 44*(11), 978-996.

U.S. Food and Drug Administration (2007). Antidepressant use in children and adults: Revisions to medication guide. http://www.fda.gov/Drugs/DrugSafety/Informationby DrugClass/ucm096273.htm retrieved on 3/1/11

U.S. Food and Drug Administration (2008, January 31). Information on carbamazepine (marketed as carbatrol, equetro, tegretol, and generics) with FDA alerts. http:www.fda.gov/Drugs/DrugSafety/PostmarketDrugSafetyInformationfor PatientsandProviders/ucm10784.htm retrieved on 3/1/11

U.S. Food and Drug Administration (2009, January). Highlights of prescribing information. http://www.fda./downloads./AdvisoryCommittees/CommiteesMeetingMaterials/Pediatr ic Advisory/Committee/UCM166792.pdf retrieved on 12/22/11

U.S. Department of Health and Human Services (2007). The AFCARS Report. Retrieved on September 12, 2008, from http://www.acf.dhhs.gov/programs/cb/stats_research/alcars/ tar/report13.htm

Vieta, E., and Suppes, T. (2008). Bipolar II disorder: Arguments for and against a distinct diagnostic entity. *Bipolar Disorders, 10,* 163-178.

Watch List (Producer) and Shoshana Guy (Producer). (2011-January 7). The Medication of Children in Foster Care (DVD). www.pbs.org/wnet/need-to-know/health/video-the-watch-list-the-medication-of-foster-children/6232

Weiss, S. R.B., Clark, M., Rosen, J. R., Smith, M. A., and Post, R. M. (1995). Contingent tolerance in the anticonvulsant effects of carbamazepine: Relationship to loss of endogenous adaptive mechanisms. *Brain Research Reviews, 20,* 305-325.

Whitaker, R. (2010). *Anatomy of an epidemic.* New York: Crown Publishers.

Wicki, W., and Angst, J. (1991). The Zurich study: X. Hypomania in a 28-30 year-old cohort. *European Archives of Psychiatry and Clinical Neuroscience, 240,* 339-348.

Winokur, G., Clayton, P. J., and Reich, T. (1969). *Manic Depressive Illness.* St. Louis: C.V. Mosby Company.

Winocur, G., Coryell, W., Akiskal, H.S., Endicott, J., Keller, M., and Mueller, T. (1994). Manic-depressive (bipolar) disorder: the course in light of a prospective ten-year follow-up of 131 patients. Acta Psychiatrica Scandanavia, 89 (2), 102-110.

Woods, S. W., Martin, A., Spector, S. G., and McGlashan, T. H. (2002). Effects of development on olanzapine-associated adverse events. *Journal of the American Academy of Child and Adolescent Psychiatry, 41* (12), 1439-1446.

Wozniak, J., Biederman, J., Mundy, E., Mennin, D., and Faraone, S. V. (1995). A pilot family study of childhood-onset mania. *Journal of the American Academy of Child and Adolescent Psychiatry, 34,* 1577-1583.

Zarate, C. A., Tohen, M., Land, M., and Cavanagh, S. (2000). Functional impairment and cognition in bipolar disorder. *Psychiatric Quarterly, 71* (4), 309-329.

Zhang, H., Du, M., and Zhuang, S. (2010). Impact of long-term treatment of methylphenidate on height and weight of school age children with ADHD. *Neuropediatrics, 41* (2), 55-59.

Ziv, Y., and Schwartz, M. (2008). Immune-based regulation of adult neurogenesis: Implications for learning and memory. *Brain, Behavior, and Immunity, 22,* 167-176.

March 2004 FDA issues Public Health Advisory on cautions for the use of antidepressants in adults and children. www.fda.gov/bb/topics/ANSWERS/ 2004/ANS01283.html

In: Child Welfare
Editors: Alex Powell and Jenna Gray-Peterson

ISBN: 978-1-62257-826-9
© 2013 Nova Science Publishers, Inc.

Chapter 3

PROTECTING THE PROTECTORS: SECONDARY TRAUMATIC STRESS IN CHILD WELFARE PROFESSIONALS

Ginny Sprang[1], Carlton Craig[2] and James J. Clark[2]
[1]Child Welfare and Children's Mental Health, Center on Trauma and Children, University of Kentucky, Lexington, Kentucky, US
[2]University of Kentucky, Center on Trauma and Children, Kentucky, US

ABSTRACT

This chapter provides an overview of a study that investigates predictors of STS in a national sample of 669 professionals, highlighting and exploring the differential responses of child welfare workers. Study participants were recruited via licensure board rosters and professional membership lists in six states, and invited to participate in an online survey.

All participants completed the Professional Quality of Life IV (Stamm, 2000). Findings indicate that child welfare job status, religious participation and rurality predicted higher levels of STS and Burnout in the sample. Comparisons of STS and Burnout among the other professions were nonsignificant. Strategies for improving worker self-care, and organizational approaches towards STS prevention, early intervention and treatment for child welfare agencies are provided.

INTRODUCTION

In 2003, the Child Welfare League of America, upon request of Congress and the U.S. General Accounting Office, issued a report detailing the challenges confronting child welfare workers in the United States. This report underscores the realities of child protection work in this country and how factors such as large caseloads, workplace stress, and worker attrition can ultimately and negatively impact the safety and well-being of maltreated children. This report stops short of identifying the types of workplace stress that may impact child welfare workers, largely due to a lack of available data to explicate the prevalence and types of stress in the child welfare milieu. However, a decade of research reveals the harmful consequences to a worker's sense of well-being and effectiveness that may manifest as a result of exposure to the recounting of traumatic, maltreatment experiences by clients. Secondary Traumatic Stress (STS) has been described as a typical "occupational hazard" that may result from certain types of work experiences (Hopkins, Cohen-Callow, Kim and Hwang, 2010; Van Hook, and Rothenberg, 2009; Conrad, Kellar-Guenther, 2006). Unfortunately, just how child welfare workers' experiences may impact the development of STS and other forms of occupational stress and how these conditions might differ across professions is not well-established in the literature. Despite such limited knowledge, the menu of approaches to preventing and treating STS are universally applied to all workers, as if the needs and experiences across professional groups are identical.

This chapter examines predictors of secondary traumatic stress, and burnout in a national sample of helping professionals, with a specific focus on the unique responses of child welfare workers. The inclusion of different professional groups in the investigation of these conditions allows for comparisons to be made across groups, and distinctions in response strategies specific to child welfare workers to be crafted accordingly.

LITERATURE REVIEW

Over the past few years, literature has emerged that suggests that the nature of child protection work may produce increased risk for the development of secondary traumatic stress in child welfare professionals (Dane, 2000; Pryce, Shackelford and Pryce, 2007). Pearlman and Saakvitne (1995) state that "graphic descriptions of violent events, realities of people's cruelty to one another, and trauma-related re-enactments" (p.31) can be harmful experiences and those exposed may develop psychological distress as a natural consequence. Indeed, this type of exposure is a common experience for who perform daily tasks that involve interviewing children about the violence and maltreatment experiences they have endured, case briefings that chronicle cruel and abusive childhood experiences, and confrontations with parents who are physically and emotionally threatening.

Secondary traumatic stress is defined as the presence of symptoms of Post-traumatic Stress Disorder, which is expressed by symptoms clustering around the domains of avoidance, re-experiencing, and/or increased arousal. These symptoms are precipitated by exposure to traumatic material indirectly, usually through the recounting of trauma experiences by clients or patients. STS is distinguished from burnout, which is also work-related, but not linked to direct or indirect exposure to traumatic material. The term Compassion Fatigue was used by Charles Figley (1995) in an attempt to describe the phenomenon in a less stigmatizing manner. Vicarious Trauma refers to the process of disruption in one's sense of safety, control, trust, intimacy, and trust as a result of cumulative exposure to traumatic material over time (Pearlman and Saakvitne, 1995). Burnout is thought to be the result of more benign, yet stressful occupational conditions such as long hours, poor organizational support and/or overwhelming workload, but is not related to trauma exposure per se. Symptoms of burnout include withdrawal and avoidance, characterized by emotional exhaustion, depersonalization and reduced feelings of personal accomplishment.

A few studies have examined child protection workers' experiences with work-related distress. Conrad and Kellar-Guenther (2006) examined 363 child protection case workers and supervisors in Colorado and found that almost 50% of child protection caseworkers had "high" or "extremely high" risk of compassion fatigue, while only 7.7% reported "high" or "extremely high" risk of burnout. These findings raise questions about why risk would be so high for compassion fatigue and so low for burnout in this group of child welfare professionals.

Van Hook and Rothenburg (2009) examined compassion fatigue, and burnout in a sample of 175 child welfare workers in Central Florida. Findings revealed higher levels of compassion fatigue (mean = 15.2) ; more for female workers and younger workers; and slightly higher levels of burnout (mean = 23.1), than the average reported by Stamm (2005), based on national norms from mixed professional group respondents.

Job focus and population-specific factors have also been found to predict variations in secondary traumatic stress in a number of studies. Ben-Porat and Itzhaky (2009) in a study of social workers employed at domestic violence shelters and child welfare agencies found moderate secondary traumatic stress symptoms in family violence workers when compared to professionals working with other victim groups. This suggests that event-specific characteristics may predict of STS, following a path similar to how the types of exposures impact the development of PTSD. A study by Perron and Hitlz (2006) examined the impact of task execution on the level of secondary traumatic stress and burnout in child welfare investigators. In this study, the authors examined the difference in mean burnout and secondary trauma scores by percentage of work directly related to forensic interviewing. Subjects who stated that 75–100% of their work is directly related to forensic interviewing scored slightly higher on the disengagement score, but no differences on exhaustion or secondary trauma scores. This finding provides only modest support for the proposal that a high proportion of work directly related to forensic interviewing is associated with secondary traumatic stress or aspects of burnout such as exhaustion.

Cornille and Meyers (1999) found 37% of child welfare respondents in their study were experiencing clinical levels of emotional distress associated with secondary traumatic stress, with levels of work exposure and work-related personal trauma predicting the presence of STS symptoms. A subsequent study by these same researchers examined self-report data on 205 child welfare workers in one southern state. Overall symptoms of workers as determined on the Brief Symptom Inventory were at higher rates on this measure of more generalized psychological distress than for the general population, and at lower rates than for a population of persons in outpatient psychotherapy (Meyers and Cornille, 2002).

There is a paucity of research exploring associations between a helping professional's sense of spirituality/religious participation or beliefs, and the development of symptoms of distress related to occupational functioning. However, Pearlman and Saakvitne (1995) note that a professional's quality of life may be associated with the professional's belief system. They note that professionals with a "larger sense of meaning and connection" are less likely to experience symptoms of vicarious trauma (p. 161). A survey conducted by the American Counseling Association indicates that counselors view spirituality as an important component of mental health (Graham, Furr, Flowers, and Burke, 2001). These authors found a positive relationship between religion and spirituality in coping with stress as well as spiritual health and immunity to stressful situations (Graham et al., 2001). Simpson's (2006) study of counseling professionals noted that higher levels of spirituality were negatively correlated with compassion fatigue, indicating that as spirituality decreases the likelihood of compassion fatigue increases. This study highlighted the importance of internal coping resources as protective factors against occupational stress and secondary traumatic stress responses.

Conversely, Roberts, Flannelly, Weaver, and Figley (2003) studied compassion fatigue among 317 chaplains, clergy and other respondents after the September 11th, 2001 terrorist attacks. Factors such as workplace proximity to Ground Zero, religion, and length of time volunteering for a relief agency had no effect on compassion fatigue. Simarly, Udipi, Veach, Kao, and LeRoy (2008) found use of religion to cope with stress (based on items from the BriefCOPE) as a predictor of higher risk for secondary traumatic stress, and as a correlate of burnout. It is noteworthy, however, that none of these studies investigated religious activity as a predictor of burnout or secondary traumatic stress in child welfare workers.

In recent years, a modest amount of literature has emerged that documents predictors of secondary traumatic stress and burnout in various subgroups of helping professionals. Studies Ting, Jacobsen, Sanders, Bride, and Harrington, 2005; Craig and Sprang, 2010; Eastwood and Ecklund, 2008; Meldrum, King, and Spooner, 2002 document that from 6% to 53% of behavioral health therapists, are at high risk for developing secondary traumatic stress. This risk is also noted for 28% - 40% of emergency workers (Hooper, Craig, Janvrin, Wetzel, and Reimels, 2010; Wee and Myers, 2003; Wee and Myers, 2002), and up to 31% of substance use counselors (Bride, Hatcher, and Humble, 2009; Adams and Riggs, 2008). Considering burnout, studies document 12 -19% of therapists (Steed and Bicknell, 2001; Craig and Sprang, 2010;), and 26% -37% of emergency response personnel (Hooper et al, 2010; Musat and Hamid, 2008) report symptoms of emotional exhaustion.

Based on this literature, it appears that any professional who has sensory exposure to distressing material (direct or indirect) and is in a work-environment with high organizational demands and low resource allocation is at risk of secondary traumatic stress and/or burnout. However, risk increases for certain employees. Females, individuals who score high in professional empathy, those with a history of prior trauma exposure, workers with large caseload of traumatized clients, and those who are socially or organizationally isolated, or feel professionally compromised due to inadequate training (Sprang, Whitt-Woosley, and Clark, 2007; Bride, Hatcher, and Humble, 2009) are at most risk. Factors such as more years of professional experience, a regular practice of self-care, and the use of evidence-based practices (Craig and Sprang 2010) have been found to be protective against the development of secondary traumatic stress and burnout.

Unfortunately, the current research knowledge base provides little direction regarding what variables might affect the development of secondary traumatic stress and burnout in child welfare workers. Our study expands the understanding of how professional status impacts the development of occupational distress by specifically including work type in the predictive model and by looking beyond 'within-group only' variations.

METHODS

A sample of professionals were recruited from New York, Florida, California, Texas, Arizona, Toronto, Kentucky, Toronto, Canada, Mexico City, and Ciudad Juarez, Mexico during a six month period in 2009. These sites were selected because they met criteria for having a large number of pediatric deaths in the year proceeding data collection. Study respondents were sent email and standard mail invitations to participate to their home addresses that were obtained from purchased certification and licensing board rosters for social work, psychology, and marriage and family therapy. In addition, electronic invitations were broadcasted via professional organizations listservs and newsletters following approval from their governing boards (when applicable). Of the 23 organizations queried, three declined to direct mail their membership but posted an invitation to participate in membership mailings. Survey Monkey was used to administer the online survey, and drew responses from 668 professionals. Each survey began with an IRB approved informed consent for participation. A waiver of signed consent was obtained so that participants who consented to the study were automatically routed to the next set of questions; those who declined participation were allowed to exit the survey. An initial screening question linked respondents to survey items based on whether or not they had provided intervention services to trauma-exposed individuals. Those who responded affirmatively were administered the STS and burnout measures, regardless of the type of trauma exposure. All survey completers were offered a $10 incentive for completing the survey. Identifying information related to incentive payment was solicited from an unlinked, separate form to ensure anonymity.

Measures

Demographics. Respondents Participants were asked to identify their living location as urban (apartment), urban (single-family dwelling), suburb (apartment), suburb (single-family dwelling), rural (apartment), rural (single-family dwelling). For subsequent analyses, this variable was collapsed to urban, suburban and rural. Frequency of participation in religious activities included the response categories of (none, sporadic, active (2-3 times a month), very active (weekly or more often). The job type choices included licensed or certified child welfare workers (Bachelor and Masters level, all job types), inpatient behavioral health professionals (all types, nonmedical), outpatient behavioral health professionals (all types, nonmedical), school based psychologists and social workers, and psychiatrists). Respondents were also queried regarding their age, gender, and race.

The *Professional Quality of Life – R-IV (ProQOL)was used to measure compassion fatigue and burnout. The ProQOL* tool that measures risk of compassion fatigue and risk of burnout. According to Stamm (2005), the ProQOL operationally defines compassion fatigue as work-related trauma that may be a combination of both primary and secondary trauma. The ProQOL is a 20-item self-report that taps the frequency of symptoms on a five-point likert scale from never (1) to very often (5). Higher scores indicate the respondent is at higher risk for secondary traumatic stress or burnout. Internal consistency has been established with this measure (alpha subscale scores range from .72 (burnout) to .80 (compassion fatigue) and is widely used in the literature.

Sample

The study sample consisted of participants who were primarily white (471/76.3%), females (449/67.2%), and averaging just over 40.(SD = 11.2) years of age.

Table 1. Descriptive Statistics for Sample of Professionals

	N	F	%
Race	617		
Caucasian		471	76.3
African American		51	8.3
Asian		22	3.6
Hispanics		73	11.8
Living Location	621		
Urban		338	54.4
Suburban		195	31.4
Rural		88	14.2
Gender	627		
Males		178	28.4
Females		449	71.6
Religious Participation	621		
None		213	34.3
Very Active		125	20.1
Active		85	13.7
Sporadic		198	31.9
Job Type	630		
Child Welfare		144	22.9
Inpatient		24	3.8
Psychiatrist		106	16.8
Outpatient		224	35.6
School Based		132	21.0

Note. Percentage may not total 100% due to rounding error.

Almost 50% of respondents stated they lived in a city/urban dwelling (338/54.4%) and 34.3% reported that they did not participate in any religious activities. Outpatient mental health workers made up 35.6% of the sample, child welfare workers were 22.9% of the respondent group, and almost one third (32.2%) of the sample were child welfare workers. Missing data was low on predictor variables (age = 5.5%; race= 6%); (see Table 1). List wise deletion of missing data was used for categorical variables, which resulted in a final sample of 577 for subsequent multivariate analysis.

PASS software was used to conduct post hoc power analyses (Hintze, 2005) for all bivariate analyses and regression models using the correlation residual method. All models were found to have sufficient power (over .99 and both regression equations were found to have power over .90) with a sample of 577.

Sample

The sample was predominately Caucasian 471 (76.3%) and female 449 (67.2%) averaging 40.8 (SD = 11.2) years of age. Over half of the sample reported that they lived in a city/urban dwelling 338 (54.4%) and 213 (34.3%) of the individuals reported that they did not participate in any religious activities. Well over half the participants were either outpatient mental health workers 224 (35.6%) or child welfare workers 144 (22.9%) and 57 (32.2%) of the male sample were child welfare workers. Missing data for the predictor variables ranged from 37 (5.5%) for the age variable to 51 (7.6%) for the race variable (see Table 1 for the sample sizes of each variable). Because the variables with the most missing data were categorical variables, list wise deletion was used for missing data resulting in a final sample size of 577 for the regression models.

Power Analysis

Post hoc power analyses were conducted using PASS software (Hintze, 2005) for all bivariate analyses and for the regression models using the correlation residual method. All bivariate models were found to have sufficient power over .99 and all three regression equations were found to have power over .90. A sample of 577 was able to detect a slope change of .01 when the correlation between the independent and the dependent variables was .20. Therefore, it is reasonable to believe with high confidence that the chance of type 2 error was very minimal for these analyses.

RESULTS

Compassion fatigue (M = 14.85, SD = 12.21) and burnout (M = 17.48, SD = 5.77) were the dependent variables in the analyses. Due to being positively and significantly skewed, square root transformations were performed on the compassion fatigue (M = 3.49, SD = 1.64) variable. The square root transformation of compassion fatigue resulted in the transformed compassion fatigue variable being significantly correlated with burnout (r = .64).

Independent t-tests and one-way ANOVA analyses were conducted using gender, race, living location, religious activity and job type of behavioral health care workers. T-tests for gender revealed that males reported significantly higher levels of compassion fatigue than females. One-way ANOVA analysis with post hoc Tamhame tests that assume unequal variances revealed a significant difference for Hispanics when compared to white professionals. No other differences were found for race on compassion fatigue. Post hoc tests revealed that professionals living in rural settings were significantly more likely to report compassion fatigue than were those who lived in urban and suburban dwellings. For the religious activity variable, those who reported no religious activity reported significantly higher compassion fatigue scores than did those in the very active, active, and sporadic activity groups. An important finding for the type of job was that child welfare workers were significantly ($p < .001$) more likely to report compassion fatigue than all other types of behavioral health jobs with no differences found between the other job types. Because age was being used as a continuous variable, correlational analysis with compassion fatigue was conducted and revealed that age was significantly ($p < .001$) negatively correlated (r = -.31), suggesting that as compassion fatigue increases, age decreases in study respondents. Table 2 displays means, standard deviations and significance tests for all bivariate means testing.

Table 2. Means, Standard Deviations, t-tests, F-tests and Significance Values for the Square Root of Compassion Fatigue as the Dependent Variable

Predictors		M	SD	t
p				
Gender				
	Female	3.35	1.45	-4.72
<.0005	Male		4.07	1.82
			F	*p*
Living Situation				
	City	3.53	1.53	7.02
.001				
	Suburb	3.36++	1.55	
	Rural	4.12*	1.86	
Race				
	White	3.43	1.53	5.52
.001				
	Black	4.08	1.96	
	Asian	4.01	1.75	
	Hispanic	4.02*	1.66	
Religious Participation				
	None	4.28	1.77	26.06
<.0005				
	Very Active	3.01***1.29		
	Active	3.07***1.27		
	Sporadic	3.33***1.41		
Job Type				
	Child Welfare	4.96	1.55	47.79
<.0005				
	Inpatient	3.59** 1.73		
	Psychiatrist	2.91***1.35		
	Outpatient	3.13***1.33		
	School based	3.24***1.36		

Note: Significance for post hoc Tamhane tests   * $p < .05$. ** $p < .01$. *** $p < .001$.

  All asterisks are compared to the first group.

  ++ $p < .01$ for comparison of rural with suburb dwellers.

Burnout

  T-tests for gender revealed that men reported significantly higher rates of burnout than did women. African Americans and Asians reported significantly higher rates of burnout than Caucasian professionals.

Table 3. Means, Standard Deviations, t-tests and Significance Indicators for Burnout as the Dependent Variable

Independent p		M	SD	t
Gender				
	Female	16.71	5.65	-6.83
<.0005	Male		19.51	5.83
				F
p				
Living Situation				
	City	17.81	5.73	3.21
.04				
	Suburb	16.79	5.54	
	Rural	18.52	6.64	
Race				
	White	17.02	5.83	5.81
.001				
	Black	19.57*	5.86	
	Asian	20.50*	5.22	
	Hispanic	18.41	5.63	
Religious Participation				
	None	19.78	5.97	21.04
<.0005				
	Very Act.	15.08***	4.57	
	Active	16.78***	5.00	
	Sporadic	16.99***++	5.81	
Job Type				
	Child Welfare	21.60	5.67	26.17
<.0005				
	Inpatient	17.13*	5.88	
	Psychiatrist	16.25***	5.20	
	Outpatient	16.26***	5.26	
	School based	16.50***	5.44	

Note: Significance for post hoc Tamhane tests * p < .05. ** p < .01. *** p < .001.
All asterisks are compared to the first group.
++ p < .01 for comparison of sporadic and very active religious activity.

No other differences between racial groups for burnout were found. Professionals who were very active, active, and sporadic were significantly less likely to report burnout than were professionals who reported no religious activity. Also, individuals in the very active category had significantly less burnout than did those in the sporadic religious activity group. Only child welfare workers reported significantly higher burnout ($p < .001$) than all other workers. There were no other differences between inpatient, psychiatrists, outpatient, and school based professionals. A correlational analysis revealed a negative correlation between age and burnout ($r = -.29$, $p < .001$) suggesting that as age decreases, rates of burnout increase (see Table 3 for details of bivariate analyses).

Regression Models

Hierarchical regression models were employed to determine if the addition of geographical living location (urban, suburban, rural), participation in religious activities (none, very active, active, and sporadic) and job status of behavioral health providers (child welfare, inpatient outpatient, school based, and psychiatrists) improved prediction of compassion fatigue, and burnout above and beyond that afforded by differences in three demographic variables (i.e., gender, race, and age). Analysis was performed with IBM SPSS version 19 using SPSS Regression and SPSS Frequencies for evaluation of assumptions.

These results led to transformation of the compassion fatigue variable to reduce skewness, reduce the number of outliers, and improve the normality, linearity, and homoscedasticity of residuals. This transformation did significantly correct the skewness of the variable. A square root transformation was attempted with burnout but it resulted in a negative skew; therefore, the decision was made to not transform burnout. As for the independent variables, age was slightly skewed positively but the transformation resulted in negative skew; therefore, no transformation was made for age. With the use of a $p < .001$ criterion for Mahalanobis distance, no outliers or suppressor variables were identified.

Correlations of the dependent variables with the independent variables revealed that correlation between burnout and the predictor variables ranged from -.02 for inpatient workers to .39 for child welfare workers ($p < .001$). For square root of compassion fatigue, the correlations with the predictor variables ranged from being 0 and not significant (inpatient) to being highly significant ($r = .49$, $p < .001$) for child welfare workers. A review of the correlations of the predictor variables with each other revealed a number of significant correlations but none exceeded .45; therefore, threats of multicollinearity and singularity were eliminated.

Square Root of Compassion Fatigue

Table 4 displays the unstandardized regression coefficients (B), the standard error, the standardized regression coefficients (β), R, R2, adjusted R2, and indicators of individual predictor significance after entry of all six independent variables. R was significantly different from zero at the end of each step.

After step four, with all independent variables entered into the equation, $R = .58$, $F(14, 562) = 20.67$, $p < .001$. After step 1, with gender, race, and age in the equation, $R^2 = .15$, F_{inc} $(5, 571) = 20.21$, $p < .001$. After step 2, with living location added to prediction of square root of compassion fatigue by race, age, and gender, $R^2 = .17$, F_{inc} $(2, 569) = 6.80$, $p = .001$.

Addition of living location to the equation with race, gender, and age resulted in a significant increment in R^2. After step 3, with religious activity added to the prediction of compassion fatigue by race, age, gender and living location, R2 = .23, F_{inc} $(3, 566) = 13.84$, $p < .001$.

Table 4. Hierarchical Multiple Regression Analyses Predicting Square Root of Compassion Fatigue (N = 577)

Predictor	ΔR^2	β
Step I	.15***	
Gender		.18***
Age		-.30***
Race		
Caucasian	(reference group)	
Hispanic		.05
Black		.09*
Asian		.03
Step II	.02***	
Living Location		
City	(reference group)	
Rural		.14***
Suburb		-.01
Step III	.06***	
Religious Activity		
None	(reference group)	
Sporadic		-.21***
Active		-.20***
Very Active		-.22***
Step IV	.11***	
Job Type		
Outpatient	(reference group)	
Inpatient		.04
Psychiatrist		-.04
School Based		.02
Child Welfare		.36***
Total R^2	.34***	

*$p < .05$. **$p < .01$. ***$p < .001$.

After step four with job type added to the prediction of compassion fatigue by race, gender, age, living location and religious activity, $R^2 = .34$ (adjusted $R^2 = .32$), F_{inc} (4, 562) = 24.06, $p < .001$. The addition of the job type variable into the equation reliably increased R^2.

When examining the individual predictors for the final model, gender was found to be a significant predictor of compassion fatigue, with males significantly predicting the criterion compared to females ($p < .01$). Age was also a significant predictor, with younger behavioral health care professionals reporting higher levels of compassion fatigue.

Those professionals living in a rural setting were also more likely to report high levels of compassion fatigue compared to those who live in urban settings ($p < .05$). No religious participation significantly predicted compassion fatigue when compared to those who were very active, active, and sporadic participates in religious activities ($p \leq .001$). Child welfare worker job status was significantly more likely to predict compassion fatigue than other job types ($p < .001$). The race variable was not a significant predictor of compassion fatigue.

Burnout

Table 5 displays the unstandardized regression coefficients (B), the standard error, the standardized regression coefficients (β), R, R2, adjusted R2, and indicators of individual predictor significance after entry of all six independent variables. R was significantly different from zero at the end of each step. After step four, with all independent variables entered into the equation, $R = .50$, $F(14, 562) = 13.22$, $p < .001$.

Table 5. Hierarchical Multiple Regression Analyses Predicting Burnout (N =577)

Predictor	ΔR^2	β
Step I	.13***	
Gender		.18***
Age		-.27***
Race		
Caucasian	(reference group)	
Hispanic		.01
Black		.07
Asian		.07
Step II	.01	
Living Location		
City	(reference group)	
Rural		.05
Suburb		-.07
Step III	.05***	
Religious Activity		
None	(reference group)	
Sporadic		-.17***
Active		-.13**
Very Active		-.24***
Step IV	.07***	
Job Type		
Outpatient	(reference group)	
Inpatient		-.00
Psychiatrist		-.02
School Based		-.02
Child Welfare		.27***
Total R^2	.25***	

Note. Total R^2 will not sum to .25 due to rounding error.
*$p < .05$. **$p < .01$. ***$p < .001$.

After step 1, with gender, race, and age in the equation, $R^2 = .13$, F_{inc} (5, 571) = 16.50, p < .001. After step 2, with living location added to prediction of burnout by race, age, and gender, $R^2 = .14$, F_{inc} (2, 569) = 2.92, $p = .055$. However addition of this variable did not result in a significant increment in R^2. After step 3, religious activity added to the prediction of compassion fatigue by race, age, gender and living location, $R^2 = .18$, F_{inc} (3, 566) = 10.95, p <.001 and resulted in a significant incremental increase in R^2.

After step four with job type added into the model, the prediction of burnout by race, gender, age, living location and religious activity, $R^2 = .25$ (adjusted $R^2 = .23$), F_{inc} (4, 562) = 12.16, $p < .001$ resulted in a reliable increase in the amount of variance explained.

Gender was a significant predictor of burnout, with male gender significantly predicting burnout compared to females ($p < .01$). Younger age predicted higher burnout scores ($p < .001$) and professionals who reported no religious participation were more likely to report higher levels of burnout than respondents in the other religious activity groups (very active and sporadic) ($p \leq .001$). Child welfare worker job status was significantly more likely to predict burnout than all other job types ($p < .001$). Living location and race were not significant predictors of burnout.

DISCUSSION

This chapter presents an overview of the current state of the literature regarding the predictors of secondary traumatic stress and burnout and provides an analysis of how child welfare worker status may influence the expression of these conditions. Empirical studies, such as this one, provide opportunities to identify vulnerabilities to occupational stress in the child welfare workforce so that intervention and policy implications can be developed to improve professional quality of life, and aid in worker retention.

In this study, child welfare worker status was associated with higher levels of secondary traumatic stress, above and beyond all other model predicators. This finding is consistent with other investigations of stress and STS among the child welfare workforce (Meyers and Cornille, 2002; Van Hook and Rothenburg, 2009; Conrad and Kallar-Guenthar, 2006). In 2007, a study by Dill identified factors such as "job-mismatches characterized by poor organizational support for professionals engaged in high-risk activities" (p. 182) as particularly perilous for child welfare workers. Chalane and Sites (2008) found that emotional exhaustion, low job satisfaction, and lack of personal accomplishment were identified as significant predictors of employee nonretention, even among a sample of employees who were groomed for this type of work.

Indeed, logic would dictate that professionals in frequent contact with the sequelae of multiple forms of violence against children would experience high levels of stress, and Baird and Kracen's (2004) synthesis of the extant research literature found that vicarious trauma and STS in professionals were generated by exposure to large amounts of traumatic material. However, our study contributes the additional finding that working in child welfare was a significant predictor of STS, while job affiliation outside of child welfare proved nonsignificant.

The frequency of religious participation as a buffer against STS and burnout are new findings that have some qualitative support (Dane, 2000) in the general psychotherapy literature. However no quantitative studies of child welfare professional STS or burnout that utilized the religious participation variable could be identified. This study broadly defined religious participation to include any form of formal or informal religious activity so it is possible that this variable was detecting the respondents' sense of belonging that may be functioning as a protective factor in highly stressful situations.

Of course, all empirical studies incur limitations. The sampling frame for this study was composed of membership lists for professional groups and registered professionals belonging to state boards of licensure, i.e., the study sample was not drawn from a master list comprised exclusively of child welfare professionals. Therefore, no claim of generalizability of study findings to all child welfare professionals may be made. By excluding cases listwise when faced with missing data, the researchers could have inadvertently increased the probability of biased estimates. Fortunately, the study incurred a relatively low rate of missing data (at or under 7.6%), indicating nonsystematic patterns of missing data, thus, limiting the probability of harmful bias. Data was collected with an online survey that guaranteed respondent anonymity; however, even with such safeguards in place to enhance the validity of self-report, some social desirability bias might be present. Finally, as discussed in the literature review, many variables may impact STS and burnout, so no claim can be made that our analytic models have captured all of the significant variables involved in these phenomena. For example, it is reasonable to speculate that some child welfare tasks will by their very nature expose workers to higher levels of STS than others; e.g., front-line investigators may be more likely to have frequent exposures than supervisors who do not carry a caseload.

Implications

What can be done? In their seminal article, organizational scholars J. Nahapiet and S. Goshel (1998) introduced the concept of employment "social capital" to refer to resources that are embedded in an organization that can provide the firm with an advantage in the marketplace. Rather than only looking to market conditions to explain the fate of an organization, these authors argued that the firm can utilize its inner resources to accomplish its mission and in so doing will achieve success even in hostile environmental conditions. Drawing on various theories of social capital, and especially the rational sociology developed by James Coleman (1990), they argue that cooperative relationships that form a powerful internal social network actually facilitate the organization's activities in the world. This network of relationships often involves positive affective attachments, such as friendships, that transcend the formal roles and obligations adhering to the actual position of persons in the organization. For example, a supervisor might seek the help of a worker to accomplish a task that is novel and might not be included in the formal job description of the employee. Because of the power of respect, warmth, and mutual obligation the job will get done, despite the fact the supervisee could invoke formal bureaucratic rules and refuse the task.

The reader will reflect upon how often this type of activity occurs in a single day across many networks in a successful organization characterized by a positive climate.

Alternatively, it is obvious how an organization will be limited if there are no such degrees of freedom enabled by social capital, i.e., how tough it is do accomplish complex and novel tasks when restricted only to formal, delineated lines of responsibility and authority with no recourse to friendly working relationships. But neither do such affiliative networks guarantee success. For example, some dysfunctional organizations may boast of workplace friendships among employees, but if these are not productively utilized in the service of the organization's mission, these affiliations will often inhibit functional activities. Therefore, it is important to understand that "social capital" usually refers to those structural networks defined by "shared narratives" and characterized by trust, norms, obligations and identifications combining to create measurable organizational advantages (p. 251).

A hallmark of social capital theory is that no single person "owns" the network—not even the formal "owner" of the organization; the capital is shared by all active persons in the organization and linked to its mission.

Yet, in the end, social capital by itself creates only partial advantages. In the best case scenario, Nahapiet and Goshal emphasize that in highly competitive markets we find that successful organizations use "dense social capital" (intensive and internal combinations and exchanges among employees) to create new and significant "intellectual capital." Such newly-created intellectual capital creates the organization's competitive edge as it facilitates greater successes in an ever-changing marketplace. In other words, success occurs when social capital recombines existing intellectual capital and generates the creation of new and even more efficacious intellectual capital.

What is conducive to developing the optimal scenario of dense social capital that generates crucial, new intellectual capital? In other words, what are characteristics of this type of excellence? Successful organizations are relatively stable, allowing social capital to accumulate; they create fruitful interdependent relationship networks (as opposed to fully independent workers), which widen the circle of interlocking networks; and they establish a clear boundary within which "insiders" share the unmistakable identity of belonging to the organization—a form of institutional solidarity.

These organizations demonstrate a recognizable "esprit de corps" that we associate with highly successful military squads, sports teams, rock bands, and even those inspired design teams that find themselves embedded in otherwise moribund corporations. Complex organizations (by the nature of their complexity) do not succeed or fail in a linear manner; their complexity posits an emergent and self-adapting system that will develop or regress in nonlinear pathways. Examples of this kind of successful "complexity" include Apple, Google, and Facebook, which were vaulted to industry leadership positions unimaginable a decade ago by innovative breakthroughs driven by particularly creative and driven teams. Recent examples of "complex" failure include the financial firms that proves "too big to fail" during the economic crash of 2009, and which required unprecedented and massive government bailouts. Such successes and failures represent the nonlinear and emergent nature of complex organizations that operate in highly volatile market environments.

Such organizations also can be understood as often creating effects known as "thriving at work" (Spreitzer, Sutcliffe, Dutton, Soneschein and Grant, 2005). The "thriving" conceptual framework argues that individual employees do not thrive only because of individual characteristics, abilities, or experiences. Thriving is made possible when employees bring adequate personal resources into an organization that enhance the kind of synergistic effects described previously. This line of research indicates that creating an optimal level of interdependence will be grounded in an organizational climate of trust and respect that encourages *purposeful and agentic interactions* such as broad information sharing and decision making discretion. The "resources" (or capital) produced by such workplaces include knowledge, positive affective and relational resources, and positive meaning.

This last characteristic is crucial for individual thriving. In fact, two organizational researchers who have recently conducted intensive research on knowledge workers' productivity and morale have concluded that "of all things that can boost inner work life, the most important is making progress in meaningful work" (Amabile and Kramer, 2011, p. 72). The main characteristic of a "good day" at work is when meaningful progress has been made; the hallmark of a "bad day" at work is when hard work is stripped of meaning by a toxic or ineffective supervisor.

In sum, thriving employees create successful organizations, but organizations must first create and enhance the infrastructures and opportunities that make employee thriving even possible. While this is currently a working hypothesis being tested by organizational researchers (e.g., Porath, Spreitzer, Gibson and Garnett, 2011), logic dictates that thriving employees are much more likely to demonstrate resilience in the face of workplace stressors than those who are not thriving. We also argue that conceptual frameworks grounded in organizational perspectives are extraordinarily relevant when we think about the problem of STS and burnout in child welfare workers who are embedded in complex organizations in the public sector.

And, in fact, there are important and relevant studies of public organizations that examine these issues. Boyas and Wind (2010) have recently investigated public child welfare organizations to explain the probable causes and deleterious effects of occupational stress in those systems. Following the social capital literature, they built their conceptual model using components of trust, social relations, organizational commitment, communication, influence, and organizational fairness. Their model can fruitfully be extended to understand the implications of STS and burnout and is suggestive of testable interventions to enhance the quality of professional life for child welfare professionals. This focus on organizational-level approaches is further justified by the notable, empirical work by Glisson and Hemmelgarn (1998) who found that public child welfare organizational "climates" that were characterized by low conflict, high cooperation, and high levels of role clarity were strong predictors of positive service outcomes and service quality—and remarkably, outperformed all measures of service configuration and interagency collaborations.

This approach to understanding possible sources of success that would mitigate STS and burnout moves us away from an exclusive emphasis on child welfare workers as individuals, and from reliance on only large scale studies of child welfare "systems of care." This view augments those studies by considering organizations-in-the-marketplace a unit of analysis. If we consider the above discussion as a possible starting point for developing remedies, we would argue that interventions to prevent and manage STS and burnout should be tailored to address stressors and to generate coping approaches that are specific to the special challenges of being an employee in a child welfare organization.

One line of research that is extremely suggestive in its correlations with the social capital framework has demonstrated that effective supervision can provide a "safety net" for child welfare employees (Social Work Policy Institute, 2011), especially when enacted as task assistance, social and emotional support, and focused interpersonal interaction (Barak, Travis, Pyun and Xie, 2009). Researchers consistently find that supervisory effectiveness is crucial for stemming the flight of workers from child welfare workplaces (Hess, Kanak, and Atkins, 2009; Pecora, Whitaker, Maluccio and Barth, 2000). Fortunately, there is a growing evidence base for what constitutes the effective or ineffective supervision of workers who serve children in child welfare and behavioral health systems (Neill, 2006). Because of the crucial role supervisors play in preventing, mitigating, and buffering negative worker experiences, their activities should strive to be grounded in best practices, and evidence-informed or evidence-based approaches. Eggbeer, Mann and Seibel (2007) describe reflective supervision as one such approach for helping professionals talk meaningfully with supervisors about case experiences that, if unaddressed, probably would generate STS effects.

At the same time, organizations must build on and go beyond effective supervisory processes. Enhanced communication can be generated through programs that provide employees effective psychoeducation about STS and self-care. These can be delivered in the form of "stress inoculation" as suggested by Dane (2000), or more comprehensively, by developing a "trauma-informed child welfare system" through approaches as demonstrated by the *NCTSN Child Welfare Trauma Training Toolkit* (NCTSN, 2008).

To this end they would strive to recognize the impact of secondary trauma on the workforce, and exposure to trauma as an occupational risk that comes with serving traumatized children. Effective child protection practice is then dependent upon appropriate self-care and STS management—a mission that should be *shared* by the employee and the child welfare organization. A trauma-informed organization understands that trauma impacts organizational culture in ways that are similar to how trauma shapes an individual's world view. Finally, it is the responsibility of the trauma-informed child welfare agency to translate trauma-related knowledge into meaningful action, policy, and improvements in practices (NCTSN, 2011a).

Child welfare organizations should also consider adding evidence-based practices to their repertoire of responses, especially since recent research demonstrates the buffering effects of using trauma-informed, evidence-based practices (Craig and Sprang 2010). NCTSN has vetted these EBPs and presented them for the consideration of clinicians, administrators, and policymakers through a helpful series of fact sheets that are constantly updated and available on their website (see *NCTSN Empirically Supported Treatments and Promising Practices*, 2011b). While all workers cannot be trained to be primary providers of such treatments, the development of such capacities in child welfare organizations through employed clinical specialists and/or alignment with community behavioral health partners can serve to assist supervisors and workers as they manage the STS and burnout effects of complex child maltreatment cases. Organizational fairness can be demonstrated through promoting optimal caseload mix that reduces disproportional distributions of over-exposure to those traumatic experiences that generate STS and burnout. Giving workers the opportunities to develop and control their own work-life balance can demonstrate that organizations trust employees to exercise reasonable influence and control. Organizational flexibility is especially important because of the diversity of the child welfare work force, i.e., "one size doesn't fit all". For example, young workers may have life cycle vulnerabilities to STS not experienced by more mature workers, including their significant lack of experience with complex cases. Tailored professional development programming that addresses such STS and burnout vulnerabilities may serve to prevent the personal, professional, and social costs of early exits from the child welfare field. In sum, while the field has long recognized the importance of human service management as crucial to organizational success (see Hasenfeld, 2009 and Weinbach, 1994 for excellent overviews), the emergent empirical work linking individual thriving to organizational climate and infrastructure offers fresh approaches to the design of testable, creative, and vigorous responses to child welfare workers' struggles to effectively practice (to borrow Freud's term) an "impossible profession."

REFERENCES

Adams, R. E., Boscarino, J.A., and Figley, C.R. (2006). Compassion fatigue and psychological distress among social workers: A validation study. *American Journal of Orthopsychiatry,* 76(1), 103-108.

Adams, S. A., and Riggs, S. A. (2008). An exploratory study of vicarious trauma among therapist trainees. *Training and Education in Professional Psychology,* 2, 26-34.

Amabile, T. M. and Kramer, S. J. (2011). The power of small wins. *Harvard Business Review*, 89 (5), 70-80.

Baird, K., and Kracen, A. (2006). Vicarious traumatization and secondary traumatic stress: a research synthesis. *Counselling Psychology Quarterly,* 19 (2), 181-188.

Barak, M. E. M., Travis, D. J., Pyun, H., and Xie, B. (2009). The impact of supervision on worker outcomes: a meta-analysis. *Social Service Review,* 83 (1), 3-32.

Ben-Porat, A., and Itzhaky, H. (2009). Implications of treating family violence for the therapist: Secondary traumatization, vicarious traumatization, and growth. *Journal of Family Violence,* 24, 507-115.

Bride, B. E., Hatcher, S. S., and Humble, M. N. (2009). Trauma training, trauma practices, and secondary traumatic stress among substance abuse counselors. *Traumatology,* 15(2), 96-105.

Boyas, J. and Wind, L. H. (2010). Employment-based social capital, job stress, and employee burnout: A public child welfare employee model. *Children and Youth Services Review,* 32 (3), 380-388.

Cahalane, H., and Sites, E. (2008). The climate of child welfare employee retention. *Child Welfare,* 87 (1), 91-114.

Child Welfare League of America, (2003). Child Welfare: HHS could play a greater role in helping child welfare agencies recruit and retain staff, GAO-03-357, accessed at http://www.cwla.org/programs/workforce/gaohhs.pdf March 1, 2012.

Coleman, J. (1990). Foundations of Social Theory. Cambridge: Harvard University Press.

Collins, J. (2009). Addressing secondary traumatic stress. Children's Voice, accessed at http://www.nyc.gov/html/acs/downloads/pdf/Trauma_MarApVOICE.pdf October 19, 2011.

Conrad, D., and Kellar-Guenther, Y. (2006). Compassion fatigue, burnout, and compassion satisfaction among Colorado child protection workers. *Child Abuse and Neglect,* 30 (10), 1071-1080.

Cornille, T. A., and Meyers, T. W. (1999). Secondary traumatic stress among child protection service workers: Prevalence, severity and predictive factors. *Traumatology,* 5 (1), 1-16.

Craig, C. D., and Sprang, G. (2010). Compassion satisfaction, compassion fatigue, and burnout in a national sample of trauma treatment therapists'. *Anxiety, Stress, and Coping,* 23 (3), 319-339.

Dane, B. (2000). Child welfare workers: An innovative approach for interacting with secondary trauma. *Journal of Social Work Education,* 36 (1), 27-38.

Dill, K. (2007). Impact of stressors on front-line child welfare supervisors. *Clinical Supervisor,* 26 (1/2), 177-193.

Eastwood, C. D., and Ecklund, K. (2008). Compassion fatigue risk and self-care practices among residential treatment center childcare workers. *Residential Treatment for Children and Youth,* 25 (2), 103-122.

Eggbeer, L., Mann, T. L., and Seibel, N. L. (2007). Reflective supervision: past, present, and future. *Zero to Three,* 28 (2), 5-9.

Graham, S., Furr, S., Flowers, C., and Burke, M. T. (2001). Religion and spirituality in coping with stress. *Counseling and Values,* 46 (1), 2-13.

Glisson, C. and Hemmelgarn, A. (1998). The effects of organizational climate and interorganisational coordination on the quality and outcomes of children's service system, *Child Abuse and Neglect,* 22 (5), 401-421.

Hasenfeld Y. (Ed.), Human Services as complex organizations (2nd ed.) Newbury Park, CA: Sage Publications.

Hess, P., Kanak, S., and Atkins, J. (2009). Building a model and framework for child welfare supervision. Portland, ME: National Resource Center for Family-Centered Practice and Permanency Planning and the National Child Welfare Resource Center for Organizational Improvement.

Hintze, J. L. (2005). PASS 2005: Power analysis and sample size. Kaysville, UT: NCSS.

Hooper, C., Craig, J., Janvrin, D. R., Wetsel, M. A., and Reimels, E. (2010). Compassion satisfaction, burnout, and compassion fatigue among emergency nurses compared with nurses in other selected inpatient specialties. *Journal of Emergency Nursing, 36* (5), 420-427.

Hopkins, K. M., Cohen-Callow, A., Kim, H. J., and Hwang, J. (2010). Beyond intent to leave: Using multiple outcome measures for assessing turnover in child welfare. *Children and Youth Services Review,* 32 (10), 1380-1387.

Kahill, S. (1988). Interventions for burnout in the helping professions: A review of the empirical evidence. *Canadian Journal of Counselling Review,* 22 (3) 31-342.

Meldrum, L., King, R., and Spooner, D. (2002). Secondary traumatic stress in case managers working in community mental health services. In C. R. Figley (Ed.), Treating compassion fatigue. New York: Brunner-Routledge.

Musat, S. A., and Hamid, A. A. R. M. (2008). Psychological problems among aid workers operating in Darfur. *Social Behavior and Personality,* 36, 407-416.

Nahapiet, J. and Goshel, S. (1998). Social capital, intellectual capital, and the organizational advantage. *Academy of Management Review,* 23, 242-266.

National Child Traumatic Stress Network (NCTSN). (2008). NCTSN Child Welfare Trauma Training Toolkit. Retrieved from: http://nctsn.org/products/child-welfare-trauma-training-toolkit-2008.

National Child Traumatic Stress Network (NCTSN). Secondary Traumatic Stress Committee. (2011a). Secondary traumatic stress: A fact sheet for child serving professionals. Los Angeles, CA and Durham, NC: National Center for Child Traumatic Stress.

National Child Traumatic Stress Network (NCTSN). (2011b). Empirically Supported Treatments and Promising Practices. Retrieved from: http://www.nctsnet.org/nctsn_assets/pdfs/promising_practices/NCTSN_E-STable_21705.pdf.

Neill, T.K. (2006). Helping others help children. Washington DC: American Psychological Association Press.

Pearlman, L. A., and Mac Ian, P.S. (1995). Vicarious traumatization: An empirical study on the effects of trauma work on trauma therapists. *Professional Psychology: Research and Practice,* 26(6), 558-565.

Pecora, P. J., Whittaker, J. K., Maluccio, A. N., Barth, R. P., and Plotnick, R. D. (2000). The child welfare challenge: Policy, practice, and research. (Second ed.). Hawthorne, New York: Aldine DeGruyter.

Perron, B. E., and Hitlz, B. S. (2006). Burnout and secondary trauma among forensic interviewers of traumatized children. *Child and Adolescent Social Work Journal,* 23, 216-234.

Porath, C.L., Spreitzer, G., Gibson, C., and Garnett, F.S. (2011). Thriving in the workplace: Towards its measurement, construct validation, and theoretical refinement. *Journal of Organizational Behavior*, In press.

Pryce, J. G., Shackelford, K. K., and Pryce, D. H. (2007). Secondary traumatic stress and the child welfare professional. Chicago, IL US: Lyceum Books.

Roberts, R. S. B., Flannelly, K. J., Weaver, A. J., and Figley, C. R. (2003). Compassion fatigue among chaplains, clergy, and other respondents after September 11th. *The Journal of Nervous And Mental Disease,* 191(11), 756-758.

Simpson, L. R. (2006). Level of spirituality as a predictor of the occurrence of compassion fatigue among counseling professionals in Mississippi., ProQuest Information and Learning, US.

Social Work Policy Institute. (2011). Supervision: The safety net for front-line child welfare practice. Retrieved from: http://www.socialworkpolicy.org/--content/uploads /2011/03/SWPI--- ChildWelfare---Supervision---Final---Report.pdf.

Sprang, G., Clark, J. J., and Whitt-Woosley, A. (2007). Compassion fatigue, compassion satisfaction, and burnout: Factors impacting a professional's quality of life. *Journal of Loss and Trauma,* 12, 259-280.

Spreitzer, G. M., Sutcliffe, K., Dutton, J., Sonenshein, S., and Grant, M. (2005). A socially embedded model of thriving at work. *Organization Science*, 16, 537–549.

Stamm, B. H. (2005). *Professional quality of life: Compassion satisfaction and fatigue subscales, R-IV (ProQOL).* Retrieved from http://www.isu.edu/~bhstamm.

Steed, L., and Bicknell, J. (2001). Trauma and the therapist: The experience of therapists working with perpetrators of sexual abuse. *The Australasian Journal of Disaster and Trauma Studies,* 2001(1), 5.

Udipi, S.,Veach, M. P., Kao, J., and LeRoy, B.S. (2008). The psychic costs of empathic engagement: Personal and demographic predictors of genetic counselor compassion fatigue. *Journal of Genetic Counseling,* 17, 459-471.

Van Hook, M. P., and Rothenburg, M. (2009). Quality of life and compassion satisfaction/fatigue and burnout in child welfare workers: A study of the child welfare workers in community-based care organizations in central Florida. *Social Work and Christianity,* 36, 36-54.

Wee, D., and Myers, D. (2003). Compassion satisfaction, compassion fatigue, and critical incident stress management. *International Journal of Emergency Mental Health,* 5, 33-37.

Weinbach, R. (1994). The social worker as manager: Theory and practice, 2nd Ed. Needham Heights: Allyn and Bacon.

In: Child Welfare   ISBN: 978-1-62257-826-9
Editors: Alex Powell and Jenna Gray-Peterson   © 2013 Nova Science Publishers, Inc.

Chapter 4

TRANSFORMING MENTAL HEALTH PRACTICE IN CHILD-SERVING SYSTEMS: A STATEWIDE MODEL FOR DISSEMINATING, IMPLEMENTING, AND SUSTAINING A TRAUMA-INFORMED, EVIDENCE-BASED PRACTICE

Patti P. van Eys, Jon S. Ebert and Richard A. Epstein*
Vanderbilt University School of Medicine,
Department of Psychiatry
Center of Excellence for Children in State Custody,
Nashville, Tennessee, US

ABSTRACT

Policymakers are increasingly charging public-sector child-serving systems (e.g., mental health, child welfare, juvenile justice) to implement evidence-based practices. Recent reviews reveal a relative lack of data regarding the effectiveness of specific dissemination and implementation strategies, but have identified a number of factors such as government funding and ideological support, organizational openness to change, active learning models and ongoing consultation/supervision that may be associated with effectiveness. Various conceptual models have emerged that incorporate some or all of these factors. The current chapter will begin with a review of the dissemination and implementation science literature. This review will be followed by a description of the Tennessee Trauma-Focused Cognitive Behavioral Therapy (TF-CBT) Learning Collaborative, a statewide dissemination and implementation project led by the five Centers of Excellence for Children in State Custody in the state of Tennessee in collaboration with experts from the National Child Traumatic Stress Network and community partners. Since 2008, the Tennessee TF-CBT Learning Collaborative has trained more than 700 clinicians in 50 community mental health agencies across the state

---

* Corresponding Author: Patti P. van Eys, Ph.D. Clinical Manager, Behavioral Health, Volunteer State Health Plan, 1 Cameron Hill, Chattanooga, TN , 37402; Phone: 423-535-8151, Fax: 423-535-3558, Email: pattivaneys @vshptn.com

using the National Center for Child Traumatic Stress Learning Collaborative model through four 9-month learning collaborative experiences. These intensive training opportunities were followed with six booster sessions for new staff within the agencies, six advanced topic trainings for supervisors and advanced clinicians, and ongoing consultation calls for clinicians, supervisors and agency senior leaders. This presentation of the efforts in Tennessee will be followed by a discussion of the lessons learned from the Tennessee experience that may help others overcome dissemination and implementation challenges in their jurisdictions.

I. INTRODUCTION

In his seminal article about the dissemination of innovation in health care, Berwick (2003) recounted the story of the British navy's more than 200-year long battle with scurvy. Scurvy is a disease that presents with symptoms of malaise and lethargy, spots on the skin, bleeding from the mucous membranes, and which causes death in severe cases. We know today that scurvy can be effectively treated by eating fresh food, particularly citrus fruits, because it is caused by a vitamin C deficiency. For centuries, however, scurvy was one of the main threats to naval crews, whose standard diet − due to extended periods of time at sea − did not include fresh fruits and vegetables. Although evidence demonstrating that scurvy in sailors could be prevented by using lemon juice supplements was known by the early 1600s, it was more than 200 years before the British Board of Trade adopted the innovation of providing citrus fruits to everyone on naval ships (Berwick, 2003).

Berwick's "scurvy story" suggests that the dissemination of innovation in health care has always been challenging; indeed, similar struggles persist today. Consider, for example, the ongoing battle against hospital-acquired infections. It has long been known that by washing their hands hospital employees can dramatically reduce the incidence of hospital-acquired infections (Gawande, 2007, 2009). Efforts to implement hand washing protocols, however, have met with limited success. One study, based on the observation of more than 20,000 hand washing opportunities from 1994 to 1997 at a teaching hospital in Switzerland, and designed to evaluate the impact of a hand hygiene improvement campaign reported that compliance with hand washing protocols increased from 48% to 66% over the 3-year study period (Pittet et al., 2000). This protocol was an overwhelming success, but also one that continued to leave significant room for improvement. The challenges to disseminating innovation in healthcare are not restricted to hand washing; research suggests that, on average, it takes 17 years for research evidence to reach clinical practice (Balas and Boren, 2000; Westfall, Mold, and Fagnan, 2007).

The state of affairs for mental health care in child welfare and juvenile justice settings is, unfortunately, much the same as it is in health care more generally. That is, we now know that effective, evidence-based practices are available, but much work remains to be done to disseminate and implement these practices in real-world, clinical practice settings (Hoagwood, Burns, Kiser, Ringeisen, and Schoenwald, 2001; Hoagwood and Olin, 2002). In the paper that follows, we will briefly review some of the barriers to disseminating and implementing evidence-based practices in child welfare and juvenile justice settings, discuss an effort to disseminate Trauma-Focused Cognitive Behavioral Therapy (TF-CBT) to community mental health care providers who work with children and youth in the Tennessee child welfare and juvenile justice systems, and summarize the implications of the Tennessee experience for efforts to disseminate evidence-based mental health care in child welfare and juvenile justice settings more generally.

II. BARRIERS TO DISSEMINATING EVIDENCE-BASED MENTAL HEALTH CARE

In large part, it is the unmet need for evidence-based mental health care (Ringel and Sturm, 2001) that prompted policymakers to task child welfare and juvenile justice systems to implement evidence-based practices (President's New Freedom Commision on Mental Health, 2003; U. S. Public Health Service, 2000). Ringel and Sturm (2001) reported that although 20% of all children and youth in the U.S. had a diagnosable mental health problem in 1999, only 5 to 7% received specialty mental health care. Children and youth in the child welfare and juvenile justice systems are at increased risk for mental health problems and for receiving suboptimal care (Burns et al., 1995; Burns and Friedman, 1990; Burns et al., 2004; dosReis, Zito, Safer, and Soeken, 2001; Zito et al., 2003; Zito, Safer, Zuckerman, Gardner, and Soeken, 2005). Thus, the unmet need for evidence-based mental health care in these child-serving systems is likely even greater (Hoagwood and Olin, 2002; Lewis et al., 2004).

Funding for evidence-based mental health care in the child welfare and juvenile justice systems is one, among many, systemic or structural barriers to the dissemination and implementation of evidence-based mental health care in the child welfare and juvenile justice systems (Hensler, Wilson, and Sadler, 2004; Proctor, 2012). Recent reviews suggest that other systemic or structural barriers including organizational support for the use of evidence-based practices and "attitudinal" factors such as an individual practitioner's or an organization's readiness for change must also be addressed (Beidas and Kendall, 2010; McHugh and Barlow, 2010). Consider, for example, a hypothetical residential treatment center whose standard of care is to provide one hour per week of individual therapy and one hour per week of group therapy to all of the children and youth in its program. Implementation of evidence-based mental health care that includes more frequent or longer therapy sessions may require significant changes to program structure and some organizations may be better equipped to make such changes than others.

Attempting to understand barriers and successes to implementation of evidence-based practices, Fixsen et al. (2005) describe implementation as a process that includes six stages. Basic descriptions of each of the six stages are below (Fixsen, Naoom, Blase, Friedman, and Wallace, 2005):

1. *Exploration/Adoption Stage* –the pre-implementation stage during which the idea of implementing an evidence-based practice originates and the potential fit between the practice and community needs and resources is assessed;
2. *Program Installation Stage* –the pre-implementation stage after which the decision to implement an evidence-based practice has been made and in which formal planning activities occur;
3. *Initial Implementation Stage* –the implementation stage in which formal implementation activities such as training staff and creating a referral base occur;

4. *Full Operation Stage* – the implementation stage in which the evidence-based practice is integrated into standard practice and can be considered, in casual terms, "fully operational";

5. *Innovation Stage* – the post-implementation stage in which there is an opportunity to refine and expand the evidence-based practice to better fit local contextual resources and challenges; and

6. *Sustainability Stage* –t he post-implementation stage in which effort must be devoted to continuing the hard work of the previous stages to train new staff, develop new leadership, and maintain the long-term viability of the implementation.

Other descriptions of conceptual models of dissemination / implementation describe similar stages (Aarons, Hurlburt, and Horwitz, 2011; Beidas and Kendall, 2010; McHugh and Barlow, 2010), and existing literature suggests a need for dissemination and implementation strategies that are specific to child welfare and juvenile justice settings (Aarons, Hurlburt, et al., 2011; Amaya-Jackson, Ebert, Forrester, and Deblinger, 2007; Markiewicz, Ebert, Ling, Amaya-Jackson, and Kisiel, 2006) and/or to evidence-based practices that address the sequelae of child maltreatment (Self-Brown, Whitaker, Berliner, and Kolko, 2012).

III. DISSEMINATING TRAUMA-FOCUSED COGNITIVE BEHAVIORAL THERAPY IN TENNESSEE

III.A. Exploration/Adoption Stage

The general purpose of the exploration/ adoption stage is to assess the needs of the community/region and match the need with an evidenced-based practice that can address that need (Fixsen et al., 2005). In this stage, so called "purveyors" of a best practice and key community stakeholders begin exploring the possibility of dissemination / implementation, and come to agreement about whether or not to proceed. There are many important considerations during this stage including (but not limited to) reaching agreement on the need for services, picking a practice to disseminate that can address that need, identifying a dissemination / implementation model, and developing a dissemination / implementation plan.

In the case of the Tennessee TF-CBT Learning Collaborative, there was a clear need to improve the quality of care for children and youth in the child welfare and juvenile justice systems. The class action *John B. v. Goetz* was a prominent example of this need (Tennessee Justice Center, 2012). TF-CBT had strong evidence supporting its effectiveness for members of this population (Cohen, Deblinger, Mannarino, and Steer, 2004; Cohen and Mannarino, 1996a, 1996b; Deblinger, Mannarino, Cohen, and Steer, 2006).There was also good evidence that very few social work, psychology and psychiatry training programs included both didactic and clinical supervision in the use of evidence-based mental health care (Weissman et al., 2006). Thus, it was clear that the best way to disseminate TF-CBT to community mental health providers was to establish a learning collaborative (Markiewicz et al., 2006).

Established as part of the settlement agreement for the aforementioned class action, the state's network of Centers of Excellence for Children in State Custody served as the primary purveyors for the Tennessee TF-CBT Learning Collaborative. Tennessee's Center of Excellence Network is a statewide network of five regional centers dedicated to improving behavioral and physical health services provided to children in or at-risk of entering Tennessee state custody. To establish the Tennessee TF-CBT Learning Collaborative, the Center of Excellence Network began by seeking mentorship from national experts in dissemination / implementation science and by identifying an appropriate dissemination / implementation model (Markiewicz et al., 2006; Saunders, Berliner, and Hanson, 2004).The main work of this stage was to establish and maintain broad support for the learning collaborative from multiple stakeholder groups across the state (Fixsen et al., 2005; Schoenwald and Hoagwood, 2001).

III.B. Program Installation Stage

The program installation stage includes tasks such as ensuring the availability of funds, creating human resource strategies, ensuring organizational readiness and relevant policy development, and creating referral mechanisms, reporting frameworks, and outcome expectations (Fixsen et al., 2005).These activities build the foundation for implementation. Perhaps the most important steps in the process during the stage of the Tennessee TF-CBT Learning Collaborative were the selection of the national expert consultants, development of the provider agency application process, and the selection of participating agencies.

To select national expert consultants, the Tennessee TF-CBT Learning Collaborative retained faculty members from the National Child Traumatic Stress Network (NCTSN) expert training pool. These faculty members were all authorized as official trainers by the TF-CBT developers and delivered training according to the NCTSN Learning Collaborative model (Markiewicz et al., 2006).

The application process for provider agencies to participate in the Tennessee TF-CBT Learning Collaborative included several steps. First, organizational readiness for change was assessed through provider agency requirements to commit to supplying a senior administrative leader, a metrics coordinator, a supervisor, and a cadre of therapists identified as "early adopters". "Early adopters" comprise about 13.5 percent of agency staff, act as opinion leaders, are well connected socially, and tend to influence colleagues toward innovation (Rogers,1995). Provider agencies were also required to conduct a self-study to anticipate organizational challenges in implementing and sustaining the provision of TF-CBT in their agencies. Areas for self-study included: a) Level of support from staff at all organizational levels-particularly leadership; b) Capacity to identify/screen referrals; c) Organizational commitment to ongoing supervision in TF-CBT; d) Staff turnover; e) Capacity to monitor progress toward implementation of TF-CBT (e.g., commitment to the metrics process). Finally, provider agencies were required to provide a letter of agreement to ensure their commitment to a 9-month process that included their team's attendance at each of three learning sessions, participation in monthly consultation calls between learning sessions, commitment for clinicians to carry at least four TF-CBT cases and supervisors to use a fidelity checklist in supervision and to carry at least two TF-CBT cases, participation in agency TF-CBT supervision, and assurance of an infrastructure for providing monthly metrics.

Provider agencies were selected based on the above criteria with a particular emphasis on their ability to demonstrate organizational openness to adopting evidence-based practices (Aarons, 2005), transformational leadership (Aarons, Sommerfeld, and Willging, 2011), a willingness to use metrics to monitor progress, and limited staff turnover. Selection as a provider agency in the Tennessee TF-CBT Learning Collaborative also required provider agency leadership to remove barriers and support changes throughout their system. Senior leadership was expected to attend all of the Learning Collaborative events, integrate system and practice changes within the organization, help the core team solve problems, review monthly fidelity metrics, support creativity and innovation, and promote spread of TF-CBT throughout the organization (Markiewicz et al., 2006).

Effective senior leadership was perhaps the most critical part of the Program Installation Stage. Provider agencies with designated senior leaders who had administrative power to make systemic change (e.g., ability to grant clinicians extra time for TF-CBT group supervision and consultation calls; power to negotiate with third party payers for more coverage for TF-CBT) were more easily able to overcome implementation barriers than were provider agencies with designated senior leaders who did not have the authority to execute organizational change. It was also important during this stage to resist the temptation to allow "struggling" provider agencies to join the Learning Collaborative; indeed, provider agencies with the resources, motivation, and "readiness" for change were the best targets for successful dissemination and implementation.

III.C. Initial Implementation Stage

Initial Implementation is a process that includes specific sets of activities and is marked by the point at which staff is in place, referrals begin to flow, organizational supports and functions begin to operate, external agents begin to honor their agreements, and individuals begin to receive services (Fixsen et al., 2005).This stage also includes the training and coaching of staff, and has the most empirical evidence on what constitutes high-quality training (Beidas and Kendall, 2010; Joyce and Showers, 2002).

Evidence suggests that didactic training alone is much less effective than a combination of didactic training, in-training practice and feedback, and ongoing coaching in the clinical practice setting (Joyce and Showers, 2002). Beidas and Kendall (2010) concluded that the important elements of an effective training program include active learning strategies such as role playing, coaching and feedback.

Therapist attitudes are also important. Therapists reporting more openness to using evidence based practices were more likely to engage in post-workshop consultation than those who reported more likelihood of diverging from evidence based practices (Nelson, Shanley, Funderburk, and Bard, 2012). In turn, this training variable (post-workshop consultation) also known as "coaching in the practice setting," is a training variable that makes a difference in skills being used in a meaningful and ongoing manner following traditional training (Joyce and Showers, 2002).

The Tennessee TF-CBT Learning Collaborate used active, adult learning strategies (Merriam and Leahy, 2005) and ongoing supervision that included both role playing and "coaching" techniques in the Learning Sessions and monthly consultation calls over the 9-month training period (Figure 1).

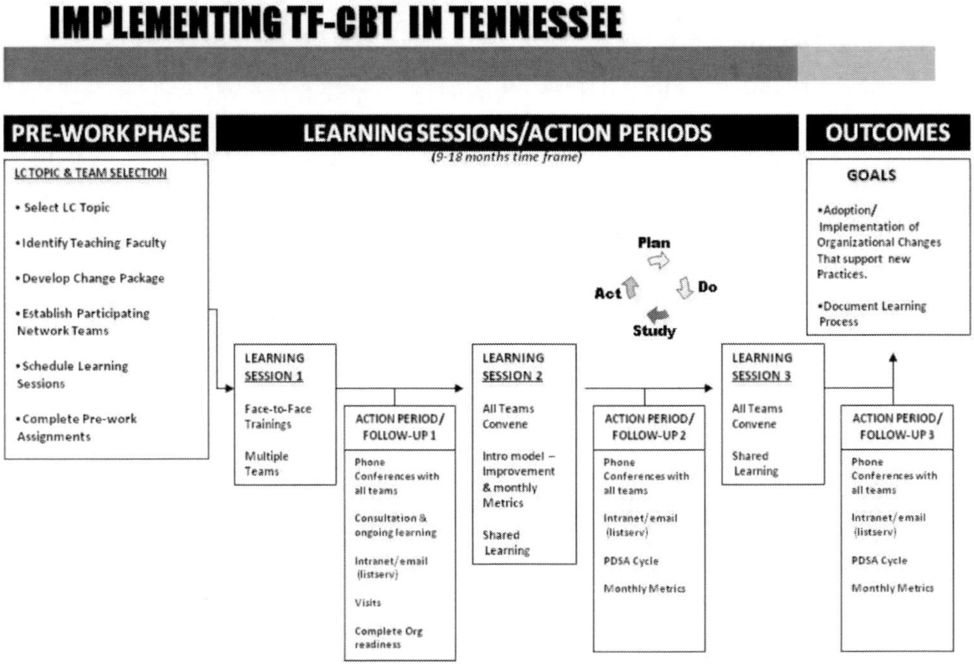

IMPLEMENTING TF-CBT IN TENNESSEE

Note: Adapted from Markiewicz, J., Ebert, L., Ling, D., Amaya-Jackson, L., and Kisel, C., (2006). *Learning Collaborative Toolkit.* Los Angeles California; Durham, North Carolina: National Center for Child Traumatic Stress.

Figure 1. Stages of the learning collaborative.

Following the NCTSN Learning Collaborative model, the Tennessee TF-CBT Learning Collaborative required purveyors, individual providers and agency teams to engage in pre-work activities, three in-person learning sessions and action periods between learning sessions.

Action period tasks included practicing new skills in the field with supervision, active "coaching," and expert monthly consultation. Throughout the process, purveyors and participants were also engaged in a quality improvement process (referred to as Plan-Do-Study-Act) which encouraged "small tests of change" for continuous improvement in the implementation process.

Along with the pre-work described above, each participant completed a web-based TF-CBT training and read the TF-CBT training manual prior to the first learning session (Cohen, Mannarino, and Deblinger, 2006). Each provider agency team also created a "story board" depicting their agency, team, and hopes for their participation in the Tennessee TF-CBT Learning Collaborative.

Pre-work for the second and third learning sessions included: 1). Creating "headlines" of success; 2). Generating developmentally sensitive and/or creative ideas for implementing a TF-CBT component; and 3). Demonstrating a quality improvement approach to addressing an implementation barrier. At the third learning session, provider agency representatives also shared a de-identified trauma narrative.

The learning sessions themselves combined didactic presentations with skills demonstration and practice. Expert faculty consultants led the learning sessions, with assistance from Tennessee Center of Excellence Network faculty. Participants provided feedback after each learning session that led to modifications in curriculum and training style, consistent with the Learning Collaborative model's emphasis on continuous quality improvement (Markiewicz et al., 2006).

One example of such a change was to have a greater emphasis on faculty demonstration of skills via role-play followed by an opportunity for participants to practice those skills and receive feedback.

This modification was consistent with research demonstrating that trainees with the highest performance in role-plays during workshops are also the ones who deliver evidence-based practices with the most fidelity in real-world, clinical practice settings (Whitaker et al., 2012).The Tennessee TF-CBT Learning Collaborative also developed an intranet to facilitate the sharing of ideas and resources between learning sessions, and also facilitated ongoing discussion and active learning between learning sessions.

The Learning Collaborative model (Markiewicz et al., 2006) also requires that critical metrics be recorded during the Initial Implementation Stage. Examples of these metrics include measures of fidelity and subsequent feedback to clinicians from supervisors and senior leaders regarding performance. To accomplish this, the Tennessee TF-CBT Learning Collaborative required provider agencies to submit information on implementation fidelity and core competencies each month.

Implementation fidelity was monitored by activities such as the number of clients receiving TF-CBT at each provider agency, the number of therapists with active TF-CBT cases, documentation of participation in TF-CBT supervision sessions, rates of completion of the TF-CBT model, and attendance on monthly consultation phone calls. Core competencies were monitored by clinicians and supervisors and measured by the completion of initial trauma assessment tools, use of specific TF-CBT components, and level of caregiver involvement.

Structured summaries of each provider agency's fidelity metrics were generated for each provider. Clinicians, supervisors, and senior leadership at each provider agency were required to review these summaries and to identify areas appropriate for improvement.

As described above, an essential element of the Learning Collaborative model is the utilization of the Plan-Do-See-Act model for quality improvement (Markiewicz et al., 2006). Provider agencies were required to make use of this model in the action periods between learning sessions to make small improvements in the quality of their implementation and to report on the outcomes of those efforts.

Critical to this stage was the impact that clinicians, supervisors and senior leaders participating in the Tennessee TF-CBT Learning Collaborative had more generally on the assessment of trauma in the state. Previously unrecognized cases had been identified and, in combination with success stories from the Learning Collaborative participants, were helping create renewed emphasis on its importance.

It also became clear that participants required more focused and direct coaching to guide a child through the process of creating his or her own trauma narrative. Thus, the Tennessee TF-CBT Learning Collaborative revised its curriculum to include a more detailed and time intensive, "step-by-step" approach to this aspect of the TF-CBT training model and the extension of an invitation to "early adopters" to share finished narratives at the third learning session. The Tennessee TF-CBT Learning Collaborative curriculum was also expanded to include advanced trainings on the topic of narrative development and processing.

III.D. Full Operation Stage

The Full Operation stage occurs when trained providers are actively taking referrals and routinely implementing the evidence-based practice with proficiency and skill. Additionally, the new services are integrated with existing services and there is full organizational and community support. Attention to solving ongoing management, funding and operational issues are notable features of advanced implementation. Fixsen et al. (2005) suggest that, on average, it takes 2 to 4 years to reach the full operation stage.

Full Operation for the Tennessee TF-CBT Learning Collaborative provider agencies began at the completion of the third learning session. During this stage, provider agencies participated in advanced coaching, supervision, consultation calls, and continued use of fidelity metrics. This meant that the "early adopter" agencies were routinely accepting clients to receive TF-CBT services and continuing to provide ongoing supervision of TF-CBT cases internally. As some participating provider agencies were reaching full operation, however, it had also become clear that others were having more difficulty. These provider agencies appeared to be those whose designated senior leader either did not have authority/support to make organizational changes and/or who had unanticipated barriers to overcome. For example, one agency had difficulty identifying a way to include caregivers in treatment sessions without leaving children in a lobby that was out of their receptionist's line of vision. This agency identified overcoming this obstacle as one of their quality improvement projects and ultimately purchased a camera that streamed video into therapist offices so that children could be both monitored and in the lobby. This agency was able to reach full operation due to its strong commitment to the implementation of TF-CBT while some other agencies were not able to overcome similar barriers to parental involvement which led to higher client attrition. It is generally thought that high rates of client attrition in treating the child welfare population can derail evidence-based practice dissemination and implementation efforts. This is a concern for a provider agency's ability to transition to the full operation stage. In the Tennessee TF-CBT Learning Collaborative, a great emphasis was placed on how to engage parents from intake through all components of TF-CBT in order to more effectively engage families and deliver more effective treatment. There seemed to be a "paradigm shift" for many clinicians from a "child in the office alone" model to an inclusion of caregivers. Also during this stage of the Tennessee TF-CBT Learning Collaborative, due to solicited participant feedback, the Tennessee faculty and expert consultants revised the curriculum to include additional emphasis on how to develop trauma narratives. Future dissemination and implementation efforts may also find it helpful to formally incorporate assessment and development of therapeutic alliance into the training process. Therapeutic alliance continues to surface as an important variable that is not an explicit focus of the TF-CBT model (Norcross and Wampold, 2011). Similarly, future implementation efforts may benefit from assessing participant backgrounds in principles of child development, family systems, and attachment in order to tailor trainings to include these pre-requisite core competencies.

III.E. Innovation Stage

The primary goal of the innovation stage is to further adapt the evidence-based practice to fit its specific local context (Fixsen et al., 2005). Although the challenge of the innovation stage is to adapt the practice to local context while simultaneously maintaining fidelity to the model, it has been noted that adaptations made after implementation are more successful than modifications made before the initial implementation is complete (Winter and Szulanski, 2001). In addition, little is known about the parameters of adaptation regarding fidelity to a model, although there appears to be merit in tailoring techniques to meet developmental stage and preference through use of flexible, creative, and individually tailored approaches (Kendall, Chu, Gifford, Hayes, and Nuauta, 1998; Kerig, Sink, Cuellar, Vanderzee, and Elfstrom, 2010).

One example of this type of adaptation in the Tennessee TF-CBT Learning Collaborative occurred in an agency that had limited resources and time to adequately provide the trauma psycho-education component to caregivers. To resolve this challenge, this agency formed parent education groups that met with one therapist for several sessions. The group format allowed this agency to provide this important psycho-educational component to caregivers without draining agency resources. The best innovations in the Tennessee TF-CBT Learning Collaborative came about when "communities" of participating provider agencies had an opportunity to exchange ideas. The intranet site provided an important online forum for this exchange. This point highlights how important it is to identify and sustain technologies for collaboration beyond the full implementation stage.

III.F. Sustainability Stage

The goal of the sustainability stage is to maintain the practice with fidelity after it has become part of standard practice and is subject to the same challenges that impact all mental health care (Proctor, 2012). Like the active implementation stages that come before it, sustaining an evidence-based practice in the community with fidelity is a process (Fixsen et al., 2005). Perhaps the best example of a large-scale dissemination and implementation project is the Improving Access to Psychological Therapies Program (IAPT Program) (McHugh and Barlow, 2010), which was backed by substantial resources and government support, provided a full-year of supervisory support, as well as ongoing didactic and competence-based training (e.g., role plays, simulation exercises). There was a substantial budget for the 3-year, active training stage (2007-2010), with provisions for additional funds to support sustainability once active training is complete.

The Improving Access to Psychological Therapies Program is a good example of how planning for the dissemination and implementation of an evidence-based practice must include sustainability. If the practice fails to be delivered or fails to be delivered with fidelity once the initial and full implementation stages are complete, then the dissemination will likely not be considered successful.

Agencies in the Tennessee TF-CBT Learning Collaborative invested clinician, supervisor, and senior leader time and purchased materials for the therapy team. Many agencies also had to alter their usual referral patterns and their usual time per client allotments in order to support TF-CBT. The goal in this stage was ensuring that providers deliver high-quality services and engaging and retaining families to achieve the desired outcomes. Very little is known about the key factors sustaining effective programs targeting child maltreatment intervention.

The Tennessee TF-CBT Learning Collaborative has been similar to the IAPT Program through the benefit of strong governmental support, that is, through state government funding. This support allowed the Tennessee TF-CBT Learning Collaborative to provide ongoing training activities to overcome some of the problems associated with staff turnover in provider agencies.

Additionally, the Tennessee TF-CBT Learning Collaborative attempted to plan for sustainability by emphasizing the need for provider agency teams to develop sustainability plans during the third learning session. Provider agency teams were encouraged to ask themselves questions such as how they would assimilate new staff into their agencies' TF-CBT culture, continue to use fidelity metrics, and provide ongoing supervision for their clinicians and clinician supervisors.

Provider agencies accomplished this in different ways. Several agencies created their own metrics, while others continued with the metrics already introduced. In addition, provider agency teams continued to have access to the intranet site for sharing of resources and ideas.

Similar to the Full Operation stage, staff turnover is an important barrier to success in the sustainability stage of the dissemination and implementation of any best practice (Aarons and Sawitzky, 2006a, 2006b; Glisson, 2002; Glisson, Dukes, and Green, 2006; Knudsen, Johnson, and Roman, 2003), even though recent research suggests that clinicians who deliver an evidence-based practice with supportive, ongoing consultation had greater 3-year job retention as compared to clinicians delivering an evidence-based practice without ongoing consultation or treatment as usual (Aarons, Fettes, Sommerfeld, and Palinkas, 2012).

The Tennessee TF-CBT Learning Collaborative found that planning for the ongoing needs of the dissemination and implementation effort facilitated sustainability. In fact, some provider agencies now claim that TF-CBT is "what we do," and in so doing has changed organizational culture (Glisson, 2002; Glisson et al., 2006). Sustainability is made much easier with ongoing financial support at the state level and when provider agency leadership willing to continue to invest real time and money.

III.G. Summary of Tennessee TF-CBT Learning Collaborative Implementation

Since 2008, the Tennessee TF-CBT Learning Collaborative trained more than 700 clinicians and 50 community mental health provider agencies to deliver TF-CBT. The planning and initial implementation were supported by partnering with national experts at NCTSN sites and the training model was based on the NCTSN Learning Collaborative Toolkit that emphasizes training clinicians in the areas of clinical competence and implementation capability in delivering evidence-based practices for trauma and facilitation of long-term sustainability of adoption of evidence-based practices (Amaya-Jackson and Derosa, 2007; Amaya-Jackson et al., 2007; Markiewicz et al., 2006).

The Tennessee TF-CBT Learning Collaborative included 9-month training experiences followed by training sessions for new staff in previously trained agencies, training sessions for experienced clinicians and supervisors, and ongoing consultation for clinicians, supervisors and senior leaders. About one-third of the 700 original trainees have participated in the ongoing training sessions.

CONCLUSION

It has been proposed that organizational systems that can effectively promote changes in staff competence, leadership, organizational supports, and the routine use of measurement performance (fidelity) will systemically position the agency to improve outcomes for children and families (Fixsen, Blase, Duda, Naoom, and Van Dyke, 2010; Fixsen, Blase, Naoom, and Wallace, 2009; Fixsen et al., 2005). Two decades of developing evidence-based practices has generated a number of evidence-based interventions for children who have experienced abuse and neglect and/or mental health problems (Hoagwood et al., 2001; Hoagwood and Olin, 2002). The current challenge is to disseminate and implement those practices with fidelity in real-world, clinical practice settings (Fixsen et al., 2009; Fixsen et al., 2005). As discussed above, several conceptual models of the dissemination / implementation process have been proposed (Aarons, Hurlburt, et al., 2011; Beidas and Kendall, 2010; Fixsen et al., 2005; McHugh and Barlow, 2010).

Although several conceptual models of the dissemination / implementation process have been proposed, the Tennessee TF-CBT Learning Collaborative found Fixsen's conceptual model (Fixsen et al., 2005) to be a particularly helpful guide for describing the process of establishing the Tennessee TF-CBT Learning Collaborative. As described above, the primary dissemination / implementation challenges encountered by the Tennessee TF-CBT Learning Collaborative of most relevance for other implementation efforts in each stage included:

1) *Exploration/Adoption Stage* – Choosing an evidence-based practice that lent itself to dissemination, selecting the appropriate dissemination model for the evidence-based practice and local context, and establishing and maintaining "buy-in" from key stakeholders across the state;
2) *Program Installation Stage* –Identifying agencies with the leadership and other organizational characteristics associated with successful dissemination, selecting and retaining national experts to augment local expertise, and developing cost effective ways to utilize that national expertise;
3) *Initial Implementation Stage* – Overcoming agency skepticism via strategic use of "early adopters" as role models, effectively using hands-on demonstration of skills practice and coaching to promote skills development, and developing mechanisms to ensure that all of the pre-work training activities are completed;
4) *Full Operation Stage* –Maintaining purveyor enthusiasm in the estimated 2 – 4 year interval between beginning initial implementation and achieving full operation;
5) *Innovation Stage* –Managing the tension between maintaining fidelity to the model of evidence-based practice being implemented and implementing innovations that will promote effective use of the new practice in the specific local context; and
6) *Sustainability Stage* – Developing plans to maintain funding for the learning collaborative activities, overcome staff turnover, and continue expanding to include new provider agencies.

Another challenge to successful dissemination / implementation that exists in some fashion in all six stages is the measurement of outcomes. The first objective is determining what the most appropriate implementation outcomes are. One typology of implementation outcomes includes acceptability, adoption, appropriateness, feasibility, fidelity, penetration, cost, and sustainability (Proctor et al., 2011). Another objective is that these implementation outcomes must be clearly differentiated from client- and system-level outcomes (Proctor, 2012; Proctor et al., 2011).In addition, because key stakeholders represent different parts of the child-serving system they necessarily have different perspectives and are therefore often most interested in client- or system-level outcomes, as opposed to implementation-level outcomes (Lyons, 2004). It has been suggested that mixed-methods evaluation designs integrating quantitative and qualitative data may help meet the need to measure outcomes at multiple levels (Aarons et al., 2012).

The Tennessee TF-CBT Learning Collaborative represents a large-scale, government supported initiative that helped change the language, practice and general culture of community mental health provider agencies and the child-welfare and juvenile justice systems' understanding, assessment, and treatment of trauma among children and youth involved in these child-serving systems. Anecdotal reports suggest that provider agencies across the state now use the language of TF-CBT to talk about these issues, screen more children for trauma-related problems, and claim to use TF-CBT with fidelity. Although these are anecdotal reports, the remaining challenge is to more formally evaluate the impact of this statewide dissemination and implementation effort. Such evidence might help support the idea that new advances in implementation science combined with strong partnerships among policymakers, mental health providers and academic partners can help further evidence-based, trauma-informed treatments more quickly and broadly.

REFERENCES

Aarons, G. A. (2005). Measuring provider attitudes toward evidence-based practice: consideration of organizational context and individual differences. *Child and Adolescent Psychiatric Clinics of North America, 14*(2), 255-271.

Aarons, G. A., Fettes, D. L., Sommerfeld, D. H., and Palinkas, L. A. (2012). Mixed methods for implementation research: application to evidence-based practice implementation and staff turnover in community-based organizations providing child welfare services. *Child Maltreatment, 17*(1), 67-79. doi: 10.1177/1077559511426908.

Aarons, G. A., Hurlburt, M., and Horwitz, S. M. (2011). Advancing a conceptual model of evidence-based practice implementation in public service sectors. [Research Support, N.I.H., Extramural]. *Administration and Policy in Mental Health, 38*(1), 4-23. doi: 10.1007/s10488-010-0327-7.

Aarons, G. A., and Sawitzky, A. C. (2006a). Organizational climate partially mediates the effect of culture on work attitudes and staff turnover in mental health services. *Administration and Policy in Mental Health, 33*(3), 289-301. doi: 10.1007/s10488-006-0039-1.

Aarons, G. A., and Sawitzky, A. C. (2006b). Organizational Culture and Climate and Mental Health Provider Attitudes Toward Evidence-Based Practice. *Psychological Services, 3*(1), 61-72. doi: 10.1037/1541-1559.3.1.61.

Aarons, G. A., Sommerfeld, D. H., and Willging, C. E. (2011). The Soft Underbelly of System Change: The Role of Leadership and Organizational Climate in Turnover during Statewide Behavioral Health Reform. *Psychological Services, 8*(4), 269-281. doi: 10.1037/a002619.

Amaya-Jackson, L., and Derosa, R. R. (2007). Treatment considerations for clinicians in applying evidence-based practice to complex presentations in child trauma. *Journal of Traumatic Stress, 20*(4), 379-390. doi: 10.1002/jts.20266.

Amaya-Jackson, L., Ebert, L., Forrester, A., and Deblinger, E. (2007). *Fidelity to the Learning Collaborative Model: Essential elements of a methodology for the adoption and implementation of evidence-based practices.* Paper presented ath te annual meeting of the National Child Traumatic Stress Network. Anaheim, CA.

Balas, E. A., and Boren, S. A. (2000). *Yearbook of medical informatics: Managing clinical knowledge for health care improvement.* Stuttgart, Germany: Schattauer Verlagsgesellschaft mbH.

Beidas, R. S., and Kendall, P. C. (2010). Training Therapists in Evidence-Based Practice: A Critical Review of Studies From a Systems-Contextual Perspective. *Clinical Psychology, 17*(1), 1-30. doi: 10.1111/j.1468-2850.2009.01187.x.

Berwick, D. M. (2003). Disseminating innovations in health care. *Journal of the American Medical Assocation, 289*(15), 1969-1975. doi: 10.1001/jama.289.15.1969.

Burns, B. J., Costello, E. J., Angold, A., Tweed, D., Stangl, D., Farmer, E. M. Z., and Erkanli, A. (1995). Children's mental health service use across service sectors. *Health Affairs, 14*(3), 147-159.

Burns, B. J., and Friedman, R. M. (1990). Examining the research base for child mental health services and policy. *Journal of Mental Health Administration, 17*, 87-97.

Burns, B. J., Phillips, S. D., Wagner, H. R., Barth, R. P., Kolko, D. J., Campbell, Y., and Landsverk, J. (2004). Mental health need and access to mental health services by youths involved with child welfare: A national survey. *Journal of the American Academy of Child and Adolescent Psychiatry, 43*(8), 960-970.

Cohen, J. A., Deblinger, E., Mannarino, A. P., and Steer, R. A. (2004). A multisite, randomized controlled trial for children with sexual abuse-related PTSD symptoms. *Journal of the American Academy of Child and Adolescent Psychiatry, 43*(4), 393-402. doi: 10.1097/00004583-200404000-00005.

Cohen, J. A., and Mannarino, A. P. (1996a). Factors that mediate treatment outcome of sexually abused preschool children. [Research Support, U.S. Gov't, P.H.S.]. *Journal of the American Academy of Child and Adolescent Psychiatry, 35*(10), 1402-1410. doi: 10.1097/00004583-199610000-00028.

Cohen, J. A., and Mannarino, A. P. (1996b). A treatment outcome study for sexually abused preschool children: initial findings. *Journal of the American Academy of Child and Adolescent Psychiatry, 35*(1), 42-50. doi: 10.1097/00004583-199601000-00011.

Cohen, J. A., Mannarino, A. P., and Deblinger, E. (2006). *Treating trauma and traumatic grief in children and adolescents.* New York, NY: Guilford Press.

Deblinger, E., Mannarino, A. P., Cohen, J. A., and Steer, R. A. (2006). A follow-up study of a multisite, randomized, controlled trial for children with sexual abuse-related PTSD symptoms. *Journal of the American Academy of Child and Adolescent Psychiatry, 45*(12), 1474-1484. doi: 10.1097/01.chi.0000240839.56114.bb.

dosReis, S., Zito, J. M., Safer, D. J., and Soeken, K. L. (2001). Mental health services for youths in foster care and disabled youths. *American Journal of Public Health, 91*(7), 1094-1099.

Fixsen, D. L., Blase, K. A., Duda, M. A., Naoom, S. F., and Van Dyke, M. (2010). Implementation of evidence-based treatments for children and adolescents: Research findings and their implications for the future. In J. R. Weisz and A. E. Kazdin (Eds.), *Evidence-based psychotherapies for children and adolescents (2nd ed.)* (pp. 435-450). New York, NY: Guilford Press.

Fixsen, D. L., Blase, K. A., Naoom, S. F., and Wallace, F. (2009). Core implementation components. *Research of Social Work Practice, 19*(5), 531-540.

Fixsen, D. L., Naoom, S. F., Blase, K. A., Friedman, R. M., and Wallace, F. (2005). Implementation research: A synthesis of the literature. Tampa, FL.

Gawande, A. (2007). *Better: A Surgeon's Notes on Performance.* New York, NY: Metropolitan Books.

Gawande, A. (2009). *The Checklist Manifesto.* New York: Metropolitan Books.

Glisson, C. (2002). The organizational context of children's mental health services. *Clinical Child and Family Psychology Review, 5*(4), 233-253.

Glisson, C., Dukes, D., and Green, P. (2006). The effects of the ARC organizational intervention on caseworker turnover, climate, and culture in children's service systems. *Child Abuse and Neglect, 30*(8), 855-880; discussion 849-854. doi: 10.1016/ j.chiabu.2005.12.010.

Hensler, D., Wilson, C., and Sadler, B. L. (2004). Closing the quality chasm in child abuse treatment: Identifying and disseminating best practices. The findings of the Kauffman Best Practices Project to help children heal from child abuse. San Diego, CA.

Hoagwood, K., Burns, B. J., Kiser, L., Ringeisen, H., and Schoenwald, S. K. (2001). Evidence-based practice in child and adolescent mental health services. [Review]. *Psychiatric Services, 52*(9), 1179-1189.

Hoagwood, K., and Olin, S. S. (2002). The NIMH blueprint for change report: research priorities in child and adolescent mental health. *Journal of the American Academy of Child and Adolescent Psychiatry, 41*(7), 760-767. doi: 10.1097/00004583-200207000-00006.

Joyce, B. R., and Showers, B. (2002). *Student achievement through staff development (3rd edition).* Alexandria, VA: Association for Supervisiion and Curriculum Development.

Kendall, P. C., Chu, B., Gifford, A., Hayes, C., and Nuauta, M. (1998). Breathing life into a manual: Flexibility and creativity with manual-based treatments. *Cognitive and Behavioral Practice, 5,* 117-198.

Kerig, P. K., Sink, H. E., Cuellar, R. E., Vanderzee, K. L., and Elfstrom, J. L. (2010). Implementing trauma-focused CBT with fidelity and flexibility: a family case study. [Case Reports]. *Journal of clinical child and adolescent psychology, 39*(5), 713-722. doi: 10.1080/15374416.2010.501291.

Knudsen, H. K., Johnson, J. A., and Roman, P. M. (2003). Retaining counseling staff at substance abuse treatment centers: effects of management practices. *Journal of Substance Abuse Treatment, 24*(2), 129-135.

Lewis, O., Sargent, J., Chaffin, M., Friedrich, W. N., Cunningham, N., Cantor, P., . . . Greenspun, D. (2004). Progress report on the development of child abuse prevention, identification, and treatment systems in Eastern Europe. *Child Abuse and Neglect, 28*(1), 93-111. doi: 10.1016/j.chiabu.2002.11.001

Lyons, J. S. (2004). *Redressing the emperor : improving our children's public mental health system.* Westport, CT: Praeger.

Markiewicz, L., Ebert, L., Ling, D., Amaya-Jackson, L., and Kisiel, C. L. (2006). *Learning Collaborative Toolkit*. Los Angeles, CA and Durham, NC: National Center for Child Traumatic Stress.

McHugh, K., and Barlow, D. (2010). The dissemination and implementation of evidence-based psychological treatments: A review of current efforts. *American Psychologist, 65*(2), 73-84.

Merriam, S. B., and Leahy, B. (2005). Learning transfer: A review of the research in adult education and training. *PAACE Journal of Lifelong Learning, 14*(1), 1-24.

Nelson, M. M., Shanley, J. R., Funderburk, B. W., and Bard, E. (2012). Therapists' attitudes toward evidence-based practices and implementation of parent-child interaction therapy. *Child Maltreat, 17*(1), 47-55. doi: 10.1177/1077559512436674.

Norcross, J. C., and Wampold, B. E. (2011). Evidence-based therapy relationships: research conclusions and clinical practices. *Psychotherapy, 48*(1), 98-102. doi: 10.1037 /a0022161.

Pittet, D., Hugonnet, S., Harbarth, S., Mourouga, P., Sauvan, V., Touveneau, S., and Perneger, T. V. (2000). Effectiveness of a hospital-wide programme to improve compliance with hand hygiene. Infection Control Programme. *Lancet, 356*(9238), 1307-1312.

President's New Freedom Commision on Mental Health. (2003). Achieving the promise: Transforming mental health care in America. Rockville, MD.

Proctor, E. (2012). Implementation science and child maltreatment: methodological advances. *Child Maltreatment, 17*(1), 107-112. doi: 10.1177/1077559512437034.

Proctor, E., Silmere, H., Raghavan, R., Hovmand, P., Aarons, G., Bunger, A., . . . Hensley, M. (2011). Outcomes for implementation research: conceptual distinctions, measurement challenges, and research agenda. *Administration and Policy in Mental Health, 38*(2), 65-76. doi: 10.1007/s10488-010-0319-7.

Ringel, J. S., and Sturm, R. (2001). National estimates of mental health utilization and expenditures for children in 1998. *Journal of Behavioral Health Services and Research, 28*(3), 319-333.

Rogers, E. M. (1995). *Diffusion of innovations* (4th Edition ed.). New York, NY: Free Press.

Saunders, B. E., Berliner, L., and Hanson, R. F. (2004). Child physical and sexual abuse: Guidelines for treatment (Revised report: April 26, 2004). Charleston, SC.

Schoenwald, S. K., and Hoagwood, K. (2001). Effectiveness, transportability, and dissemination of interventions: what matters when? *Psychiatric Services, 52*(9), 1190-1197.

Self-Brown, S., Whitaker, D. J., Berliner, L., and Kolko, D. (2012). Disseminating child malreatement interventions: Research on implementing evidence-based programs. *Child Maltreatment, epub ahead of print*.

Tennessee Justice Center. (2012). John B. v. Goetz Retrieved April 12, 2012, from http://www.tnjustice.org/resources/john-b/.

U. S. Public Health Service. (2000). Report of the Surgeon General's Conference on Children's Mental Health: A National Action Agenda. Washington, DC: Department of Health and Human Services.

Weissman, M. M., Verdeli, H., Gameroff, M. J., Bledsoe, S. E., Betts, K., Mufson, L., . . . Wickramaratne, P. (2006). National survey of psychotherapy training in psychiatry, psychology, and social work. [Research Support, Non-U.S. Gov't]. *Arch Gen Psychiatry, 63*(8), 925-934. doi: 10.1001/archpsyc.63.8.925.

Westfall, J. M., Mold, J., and Fagnan, L. (2007). Practice-based research--"Blue Highways" on the NIH roadmap. *Journal of the American Medical Assocation, 297*(4), 403-406. doi: 10.1001/jama.297.4.403.

Whitaker, D. J., Ryan, K. A., Wild, R. C., Self-Brown, S., Lutzker, J. R., Shanley, J. R., . . . Hodges, A. E. (2012). Initial Implementation Indicators From a Statewide Rollout of SafeCare Within a Child Welfare System. *Child Maltreat, 17*(1), 96-101. doi: 10.1177/1077559511430722.

Winter, S. G., and Szulanski, G. (2001). Replication as strategy. *Organization Science, 12*(6), 730-743.

Zito, J. M., Safer, D. J., DosReis, S., Gardner, J. F., Magder, L., Soeken, K., . . . Riddle, M. A. (2003). Psychotropic practice patterns for youth - A 10-year perspective. *Archives of Pediatrics and Adolescent Medicine, 157*(1), 17-25.

Zito, J. M., Safer, D. J., Zuckerman, I. H., Gardner, J. F., and Soeken, K. L. (2005). Effect of medicaid eligibility category on racial disparities in the use of psychotropic medications among youths. *Psychiatric Services, 56*(2), 157-163.

In: Child Welfare   ISBN: 978-1-62257-826-9
Editors: Alex Powell and Jenna Gray-Peterson   © 2013 Nova Science Publishers, Inc.

Chapter 5

EDUCATIONAL VULNERABILITY OF CHILDREN AND YOUTH IN FOSTER CARE

Andrea Zetlin[*]

California State University Los Angeles, Charter College of Education,
Los Angeles, California, US

ABSTRACT

Bradley, an African-American 6 year old, entered the kindergarten class in March. He had just moved, mid-school year, from across the country because his birth mother lost custody of him. While his peers were practicing writing, reading and adding, Bradley struggled to write his name. When he first arrived, the school knew only that he was in foster care and had an IEP stipulating a variety of special education services. The paperwork accompanying his enrollment was sparse because his relative caregiver was given no more documentation than the school. Although multiple school employees requested records over and over again, neither Bradley's previous school nor the school district responded to these formal requests. After several months Bradley's biological mother finally sent past IEPs and several evaluation documents that provided more insight into his school history. Just as the school was getting to know Bradley, figure out his needs, and make progress toward his goals, Bradley's biological mother regained custody and he was moved back across the country (Montreuil and Zetlin, 2012, p.3).

Students like Bradley can be found in almost every school in the nation. Children in the foster care system, like Bradley, move from school to school and home to home with a lack of consistency. The effects of this instability can be very challenging for the foster child, caregiver, school, and child welfare agency.

FOSTER CARE: FALLING THROUGH THE CRACKS?

Children in foster care number over half a million in the United States, the majority school-age. The mission of the foster care system is to protect children who have been

---

[*] Tel: (323) 343-4410; E-mail: azetlin@calstatela.edu

physically or sexually abused or neglected and reduce the risk of endangerment. Within the last decade, the child welfare system recognized the need to address educational as well as safety issues in assuming responsibility for the well being of these children. A successful school experience of children in out-of-home care can play a key role in stability in placement as well as adaptive transition out of the foster care system. However, the literature reveals that foster youth are more likely than other children to experience a myriad of academic and behavioral problems in school. Whether these educational difficulties existed prior to child welfare involvement or are the effects of maltreatment and out of home placement is still unclear. Nonetheless, research studies have found that foster children are more likely to be increasingly below grade level in reading and math the more years they spend in foster care (Emerson and Lovitt, 2003). They have higher rates of absences, disciplinary actions, and special education referrals; attain significantly lower standardized test scores; and experience higher rates of grade retention (Shea, Weinberg, and Zetlin 2011.) Scherr's (2007) meta-analysis of existing research estimated that 31 percent of foster youth qualified for or received special education services, a rate five times higher than their peers. In terms of grade retention, 33 percent of students in foster care were retained at least once during their school career and were seven times more likely to be retained than were other students. Regarding disciplinary problems, 24 percent of students in foster care were suspended or expelled from school at least once and were three times more likely than their peers to have faced disciplinary actions.

The adult outcome predictions for this population are dire with the majority not completing high school and at great risk of becoming part of the public assistance and criminal justice systems. One in four youth who age out of the foster care system are incarcerated within two years of leaving foster care. One in five former foster youth become homeless at some time after age 18. Only 46 percent complete high school; 3 percent earn a college degree; and just 51 percent have a job at age 21 (Courtney, et.al., 2011; Casey Family Programs 2003).

This manuscript will review research examining efforts by state and local child welfare and educations systems to increase attention to the educational plight of foster children. The manuscript will focus on (1) the systemic issues and barriers that put children in foster care in risk of educational failure and (2) the strategies and practices that those working with this population are implementing so that foster children and youth have opportunities to prosper educationally.

BARRIERS TO LEARNING AND ACHIEVEMENT

Three major barriers to educational progress emerged from descriptive investigations questioning youth in out-of-home care and other individuals connected to the foster care system including caregivers, personnel from school and child welfare agencies, former foster youth, and policymakers. Harker and her associates (2003) conducted interviews with 80 children and youth aged 10-18 living in foster care in England to assess their current educational progress and solicit their suggestions as to how the educational experience of those in the child welfare system might be improved. Zetlin and her associates (2006, 2010) held a series of focus group sessions with participants representing different sectors of the child welfare system in California to discuss their views on the educational problems and needs of students in foster care. California is home to almost 20 percent of the population of foster children and youth in the U.S. There is consensus across these multiple "voices" that learning and school achievement are being impeded by: placement and school instability, insufficient collaboration across the child welfare and school systems, and inadequate intervention programs and over-reliance on special education. Each barrier is described below

Placement and School Instability

The most serious problem for students in foster care appears to be the residential instability that they experience which often results in accompanying school transfers. Child protective services gives priority to meeting the abused or neglected youths' immediate physical and emotional needs with little emphasis on long-term developmental needs and educational opportunities (Harker, Dobel-Ober, Lawrence, Berridges, and Sinclair, 2003). The result is that the foster youths' homes change and their school and all the connections related to their schooling change. With each move, new caregivers and teachers are unfamiliar with the academic strengths and weaknesses of the foster youth which may disadvantage the youth educationally. Bradley's case description at the start of this chapter, illustrates this instability and its effect on the child. Harker and her associates reported that 70 percent of their sample of foster children and youth had experienced placement change with a mean of five placement moves averaging one per year. While some foster youth reported their educational progress improved when placed in care and having a safe and stable home environment, others referred to the emotional trauma of being removed from their home, difficulties of being separated from friends, and feeling conspicuous as a mid-semester arrival at a new school. They described problems concentrating at school and completing homework assignments, no one at home or school taking interest in their education or encouraging them to do well, and feeling negatively stereotyped as a foster child by the teachers and other students (Harker et.al, 2003).

Too often, transferring homes involved a delay in enrollment in the new school and extended periods of time spent out of school. For high school youth, mid-semester moves meant that the academic classes they needed were already full. They were placed in any class with an opening and sometimes fewer classes than required for a full schedule. This led to youth not taking the required courses for high school graduation or entrance to a four year college. Moreover, many foster youth who transferred mid-semester, had difficulty developing friendships and getting involved in school activities (Zetlin, Weinberg, and Shea, 2006a).

Insufficient Collaboration across the Child Welfare and School Systems

Another serious problem is the lack of communication and coordination between the school districts and child welfare agency resulting in insufficient commitment in both systems to attend to the educational welfare of children and youth in foster care. Even when school-related problems are detected and meetings arranged, because of the lack of accountability, the attitude among representatives from the school and child welfare agency too often is "it's your problem not ours" (Zetlin, Weinberg, and Shea, 2006). There appears to be no single person - caregiver, social worker, counselor or teacher - responsible for monitoring and advocating for the foster child's educational progress.

Exacerbating the lack of communication and coordination, is that each system has its own unique database and the two databases are not linked. Without a means of sharing data, the schools are unaware of which students enrolled at the school are in foster care and the child welfare agency lacks information on the academic and behavioral progress of children in their care. For schools, the effect of no shared database is intensified when a foster youth enrolls without school records. Placement in the appropriate grade, classes and/or programs is a challenge without access to the child's school records and school history.

The research revealed that too few at the child welfare agency were aware of or understood the educational problems that foster youth experienced or how to navigate the complicated school system and contact the appropriate school staff to seek help. Social workers' training did not prepare them to grasp the importance of education for children in foster care and the need for active involvement in referring foster youth for supports and services like tutoring, special education evaluation, and attendance monitoring. Within the schools, educators resented that children were moved by the child welfare agency without consideration for the impact such movement might have on educational progress and, in general, were disappointed with the level of interest and support that social workers exhibited towards education. Schools were not informed when children in foster care were transferred to a new home and needed to be disenrolled from the school's roster. School staff felt lost when dealing with the child welfare agency and figuring out, for example, who to inform when they had concerns about the foster student's performance or behavior or who had the right to make educational decisions for the child. They complained that social workers did not respond when they left a message regarding a foster child or foster parent. Further, the schools had limited resources and believed that more services could be made available for the foster youth if both systems worked as a team involving caregivers as well (Zetlin, Weinberg, and Shea, 2010.) The schools wanted the child welfare agency to require that caregivers be involved in supporting the foster child's education. School problems frequently escalated because caregivers did not show up to school meetings when learning or behavior troubles first appeared. The school believed that everyone needs to work together and responsibly do their part to help these students succeed.

Inadequate Intervention Programs and Over-reliance on Special Education

As noted earlier, students in foster care often experience a multitude of learning and behavior problems in the school setting. Moreover, too many young children in foster care are experiencing the effects of prenatal exposure to drugs including hyper-aggression, hyperactivity, and cognitive impairment. The schools and child welfare agency have few resources to identify problems early and offer prevention or early intervention programs to address learning and social skills needs, and manage behavior. Caregivers of very young children are also not required by child welfare policy to enroll their children in preschool programs.

Concerned caregivers reported seeking outside help to address their children's needs without the assistance of their social worker. They mostly struggled on their own building up their knowledge about the special education process and early intervention services and with the advice of professionals and other parents they encountered. They engaged in battles with the schools for more intensive supports often challenging the schools when their children were declared ineligible for an IEP. Social workers with their very high caseloads were not readily available to intercede if a school problem was brought to their attention. Furthermore, there were few child welfare or community resources that social workers could offer for tutoring or mental health counseling (Zetlin, et. al, 2010). .

Without the cooperation and input of the home or child welfare agency, the schools felt challenged to address the learning and behavior problems as they surfaced. Because of the lack of education supports in general education, schools over-identified students in foster care for special education assistance to obtain more intensive services. Since foster youth moved schools often, the IEPs were re-written with each new school placement and supports and services varied depending on what the new district could offer. When problems exhibited by the foster student escalated and could no longer be contained and because there was little cooperation or input from the caregiver or social worker, the schools sought more severe remedies like disciplinary transfer or placement in a nonpublic special education school. If a foster youth with emotional problems was placed in a group home with an on-site nonpublic special education school (NPS), they were often enrolled in the NPS. These schools were problematic because of low level academics, difficulty accumulating credits, not fully credentialed teachers, and limited or no extracurricular activities. Moreover, foster youth with IEPs designating NPS placement had difficulty returning to comprehensive schools (Zetlin, et. al., 2006a).

In sum, the practice and policy tensions that exist between the education and child welfare systems has led to overall academic risk for children and youth in foster care. By identifying and clarifying the barriers that impede educational progress, we can promote initiatives and adopt responsive practices to improve communication and coordination between the systems. In this way, both the education and child welfare systems will be in a better position to address proactively and collaboratively the educational challenges of this population. The next section describes some of the actions underway to improve the educational experience of students in the dependency system.

LEGISLATIVE INTERVENTION AND PROMISING PRACTICES

Julia is a 13 year old Latina youth from West County who has been in the child welfare system since her early elementary years. She has three older siblings in the system as well. Julia had been living in South County with her legal guardian awaiting adoption proceedings when her guardian withdrew from the adoption. She was fed up with Julia's running away from home, behavior outbursts, and truancy. Over the past several years, Julia was in seven schools with an average duration of one month. Julia was placed back in West County and assigned an education liaison from the West County Office of Education to serve as her case manager and advocate. The education liaison monitored Julia closely as she moved through three different school placements during the next year. Throughout this period, the education liaison worked to support Julia by arranging for a Student Study Team meeting and then assessment for special education and mental health counseling services. When Julia was found eligible for special education and then for intensive mental health services, the IEP team recommended placement in a residential school in Texas. Neither Julia's CASA (Court Appointed Special Advocate) who holds education rights nor Julia who has strong ties to her siblings wanted out of state or residential placement. The education liaison negotiated having Julia transferred to the elementary school district which she attended before her move to South County. She gathered all Julia's school records that were scattered across her previous schools and delivered them to her new school.

Beside placement in special education, Julia was placed in a therapeutic afterschool program. Julia remained stable for that whole school year and her home placement was stable as well. Then her foster father died and she was moved to a new placement. Shortly after, her new foster parent had a heart attack and Julia had to change home placements again. At this time, she graduated from 6th grade and had to move schools to attend 7th grade in the local junior high school.

This past school year, she has been regularly attending school and appears to be doing relatively well in her special education placement with supportive services. She still has occasional behavior outbursts but nothing as severe as in the past.

Since returning to West County, Julia has a strong cohesive team working for her. The education liaison continues to monitor her and is currently working to arrange one on one tutoring at her school. Her CASA checks in regularly with the school and her social worker is actively involved with the case. Through Julia's ups and downs since returning to West County, the education liaison has been an important and stable figure in her life and stepped in to assist and support Julia as needed.

Legislative Advances

Over the past two decades, federal and state legislation have been enacted to provide impetus and support for the ways the child welfare and education systems respond to the educational needs of children and youth in foster care.

The McKinney-Vento Homeless Assistance Act passed in 1987 addresses the issue of school stability. The measure focuses on homeless children which includes some children in foster care who are living in emergency shelters, awaiting foster care placement, or unaccompanied youth (i.e., runaways).

A key provision of the act is to keep homeless students enrolled in the "school of origin," the school they attended at the time of placement or in which they were last enrolled. Other provisions in the bill include (1) immediate enrollment in any school in their attendance area without the required documents (i.e., immunization record, school records, birth certificate), (2) transportation funds to transport the children from where they are living to the school of origin, and (3) the appointment within local education agencies (LEA; i.e., county office of education, school districts) of a liaison for homeless students to troubleshoot issues.

The Individuals with Disabilities Act, reauthorized in 2004, outlined new services for children with disabilities who are wards of the state (i.e., foster children or children in the custody of a public child welfare agency.) For children birth to three years who are involved in a substantiated case of abuse or neglect, state procedures must require referral for early intervention services. The Child Find provision of the act calls for schools to identify, locate, and evaluate children who are wards of the state even if those children do not have a stable home or school placement. To ensure a timely evaluation, the school can conduct the initial evaluation without parental consent, if, despite reasonable efforts, the school cannot locate the parent and the court has not assigned education rights to a surrogate. If the child changes schools before the initial evaluation is complete, the new school must coordinate their assessment with the prior schools as expeditiously as possible (Leoni and Weinberg, 2010).

No Child Left Behind Act, Title I, Part D (2001) provides financial assistance to prevention and intervention programs for children and youth who are neglected, delinquent or at risk. These funds are intended to (1) improve educational services so these high risk youth have an opportunity to meet state achievement standards and (2) prevent dropping out of school.

The educational provisions of *The Fostering Connections to Success and Increasing Adoptions Act* of 2008 mirror some aspects of the McKinney-Vento Homeless Assistance Act. The Fostering Connections act requires state child welfare agencies to improve educational stability for children in foster care by coordinating with LEAs to keep children enrolled in the school they attended at the time of placement into foster care. When a move is necessary, the agency needs to ensure immediate enrollment in a new school with the child's school records made available. To offset the cost of transporting children to school, federal funding is available to cover education-related transportation costs. The act also provides funding for states to extend care and support to youths in foster care until the age of 21 to encourage the youths to complete high school or an equivalent degree and enroll in post secondary or vocational school.

In 2004, California passed legislation known as *the Educational Rights and Stability for Foster Youth Act (Assembly Bill 490)* to address the barriers to equal educational opportunities for the state's foster children.

This act extends many of the provisions of the McKinney-Vento Homeless Assistance Act to all children and youth in the dependency system. School stability is addressed by allowing foster children to remain in their school of origin for the duration of the school year when their placement changes (provided it is in the children's best interest to do so.) When foster children change schools, the act requires the immediate enrollment in the new school (even if required documentation is not available) and the timely transfer of the students' school records within two business days.

A foster care education liaison must be designated by the LEA to ensure proper placement, transfer and enrollment in school for foster youth. In terms of grades and course credit, the foster students' grades may not be lowered due to absences caused by a change in placement or court appearance and they must be awarded full or partial credit for coursework satisfactorily completed at a school.

Lastly, when a school placement is sought, a comprehensive public school (rather than a restrictive community day or nonpublic school) must be considered as the first school placement option for foster youth. In the above case illustration, Julia benefitted from many of the provisions of AB 490. Her education liaison was able to argue for a less restrictive placement than the residential school recommended by the IEP team. She negotiated returning Julia to her elementary school district (her school of origin) in which she was enrolled prior to placement with her guardian in South County. The education liaison also made contact with the AB 490 liaisons serving schools that Julia previously attended and they helped to gather Julia's school records. Lastly, Julia was connected to programs and services (i.e., therapeutic afterschool and tutoring programs) to help her perform optimally in school.

Promising Practices

"It takes a village to raise a child" best describes what is required to provide the comprehensive and coordinated support that foster children need to improve their schooling experiences and outcomes. As indicated by the description of recent legislation whose provisions address educational opportunities for foster youth, policymakers and practitioners realize that the child welfare and school systems cannot operate in isolation to identify and resolve the academic, behavioral, and bureaucratic problems that impede the education progress of foster children. Roused by the legislation, the past 20 years has seen efforts by the two systems to work together, share scare resources, and take advantage of each other's respective disciplinary knowledge to overcome educational hurdles that hinder school progress and achieve more effective service delivery (Weinberg, Zetlin and Shea, 2009; Zetlin, Weinberg, and Kimm, 2004).

Interagency Education Workgroups

Interagency education workgroups have been used by local jurisdictions (i.e., counties) to bring together representatives from public and private agencies and organizations that can work together strategically to develop collaborative structures and formal procedures for addressing the education functioning of foster youth. One example of the use of an interagency workgroup was described in a study by Weinberg, et. al. (2009). Interagency work groups were formed in several California counties and included representatives from school districts, the child welfare agency, county departments of mental health and probation, the court, community colleges, and caregivers, among others. The first task of the work groups was to identify the specific educational issues that were preventing foster youth from achieving in schools.

Members of the workgroup met regularly and overtime became an important vehicle through which much of the interagency collaboration within the county happened. They accomplished such concrete outcomes as developing forms and procedures for the child welfare agency to use to notify the school district when a foster child would be entering or leaving a school, compiling a list of education advocates for the court to appoint as a foster child's "responsible adult," and initiating a memorandum of understanding so that school records could be shared across agencies (Leoni and Weinberg, 2010).

Education Liaisons

In California, most of the 58 counties have education liaisons that serve as a bridge between the child welfare and education systems for the purpose of troubleshooting education barriers and working to increase academic achievement and graduation rates. The education liaison model implemented in these counties take many forms and vary in terms of lead agency and funding sources, philosophy of change, backgrounds of the education liaisons, specific populations of foster youth targeted, how intensively they intervene with the foster youth, and level of collaboration that exists between child welfare and education systems. For example, in one county, the education liaisons are social workers employed by the child welfare agency and co-located in the county office of education.

Each education liaison works on addressing issues and resolving problems for a large number of referred cases and then closes the cases in a timely manner. In another county, the education liaisons are social workers but employed by the county office of education. They are housed in the offices of the child welfare agency and spend much of their time gathering school data to update education reports for the social workers to include in their semi-annual court reports. They also do crisis intervention and case management for high risk groups within the foster youth population.

Typically, the main responsibilities of the education liaison are to actively advocate for foster youth experiencing educational problems as well as focus on building and sustaining relationships with the school community. They track school data and monitor progress and problems for individual youth as well as for subgroups within the foster population (i.e., search for patterns such as middle or high school students' grades "tanking" at certain times of the school year, large numbers of foster youth being suspended).

When trends are detected, they work to develop strategies to counter the problem, for example, to address the problem of large numbers of foster youth not showing up for standardized testing, one county's education liaisons systematically contacted caregivers in advance to alert them to the date of the test. When requested, the education liaisons provide trainings to school and child welfare staff to further understanding about the educational needs of foster youth. The education liaisons also provide school information and resources to social workers and families. In some counties, the education liaisons sit on multi-disciplinary teams to advocate for foster youth and on interagency coordinating committees within the counties.

Results of a study that examined the effectiveness of the education liaison model in a large California county (Zetlin, et. al., 2006b) showed that having education liaisons available to social workers, had a positive effect on their practices. There were increases in the social workers' level of knowledge about educational procedures and programs for supporting academic progress, increases in their level of participation in the educational process of children on their caseloads, and increases in their documentation of education information included in the case files. Another positive result was improved math and reading achievement test scores of foster students served by the education liaisons.

Interagency Database

Efforts have begun in local jurisdictions to link databases between the child welfare agency and schools to use data to inform practice. By having access to shared data, the records of individual children and youth in the foster care system can be monitored and all relevant parties with some responsibility for a child are kept up-to-date on how he or she is functioning in school (Leoni and Weinberg, 2010). In one county in California, the foster youth database developed by the county office of education stores transcript, attendance and disciplinary records as well as standardized test scores, school history and special education status, among other information.

The system immediately notifies school districts about new out-of-home placements and changes in placement. Mostly, the education liaisons and social workers access the database for case management of individual foster youth and for preparing court reports. However, the system can also produce aggregate data of how foster students, in general, are performing in the county for reporting purposes.

Efforts are also underway in California and other states to develop statewide databases which will provide a means to monitor how these children and youth are functioning as a group and what systemic changes might be needed to improve their school outcomes.

CONCLUSION

Over 20 years ago, Jacobson (1998) stated that "the odds against children in foster care achieving success in school are great (p.42.)" The lack of continuity in their education including frequent school changes, periods of non-enrollment, no single adult monitoring their academic progress, and so forth has led to dismal school and post school outcomes. Knowing that investments in education are the most effective means to deter crime and lower incarceration rates and to reduce poverty and unemployment (Noguera, 2002), we cannot ignore the negative trajectory that too many former foster youth experience. Since Jacobson's remark, increased awareness of the educational plight of foster youth has led to supportive legislation and improvements in the working relationship between the child welfare and education systems. However, more work is needed. The child welfare and education systems must continue to find effective ways to work together to deliver high quality education that addresses the needs of this most vulnerable population of students.

Additional legislation, new state policy, and innovative programs and services must focus on such intractable issues as:

- Continued high levels of school instability
- Disproportionate rates of suspension, expulsion, and placement in special education of foster youth compared to the general population
- Low rates of foster youth taking standardized tests or having test scores recorded in school records (i.e., some foster youth change schools before test scores are received and scores are not forwarded by the former school to the new school)
- Lack of sustained attention to ensure that high school foster youth are enrolled in classes needed to meet the requirements for admission to four-year colleges;
- Lack of monitoring to determine the quality of schools in which students in foster care are enrolled (i.e., API levels, Teacher Effectiveness ratings).
- Lack of statewide or cross county policy for funding and monitoring out-of-county foster youth (i.e., the local child welfare agency is responsible for children whose birth family resides in that county but has no jurisdiction over foster children who reside in the county but whose birth family resides in another county or state)
- Inability to discern patterns and trends in school progress of foster youth as a unique population of students and develop interventions and/or policies to address identified concerns (i.e., foster youth are not flagged within state education databases to monitor such state or regional trends as disproportionate rates of suspension, expulsion, special education status, low test scores, etc.)
- Need for child welfare policies that mandate (1) preschool enrollment and (2) caregiver involvement/oversight of the foster child's schooling
- Need for continuous cross-training of school and child welfare personnel due to high turn-over rates in order to ensure that (1) educational issues are spotted and acted on early, and (2) coordination and collaboration are the fabric of relations between the two systems

Responsive policies and practices must continue to be designed to address these lingering needs and ultimately enhance educational opportunities for children and youth in foster care to achieve as they move through school. As our understanding of the forces that impede such progress grows, we must create the collaborative structures, organization, and practices including shared responsibility and shared accountability across agencies, to support the educational advancement and more positive adult outcomes for children and youth in the foster care system.

REFERENCES

Casey Family Programs (2003). *The foster care alumni studies: Assessing the effects of foster care.* Seatle: Casey Family Programs.

Courtney, M.E., Dworsky, A., Brown, A., Cary, C., Love, K., and Vorhies, V. (2011). Midwest evaluation of the adult functioning of former foster youth: Outcomes at age 26. Chicago, IL: Chapin Hall at the University of Chicago. Retrieved from: http://www.chapinhall.org/sites/default/files/Midwest%20Evaluation_Report_12_21_11_2.pdf

Harker, R.M, .Dobel-Ober, D., Lawrence, J., Berridges, D., and Sinclair, R. (2003). Who takes care of education? Looked after children's perceptions of support for educational progress. *Child and Family Social Work,* 8, 89-100.

Jacobson, L. (1998, September 9). *One on one. Education Week,* 18(1), 42-47.

Leoni, P. and Weinberg, L. (2010). *Addressing the unmet needs of children and youth in the juvenile justice and child welfare systems.* Washington D.C.: Georgetown University Center for Juvenile Justice Report. Retrieved from http://cjjr.georgetown.edu/pdfs/ed/edpaper.pdf

Montreuil, C. H. and Zetlin, A. (2012, January). The challenges of teaching children in foster care. *Council for Exceptional Children DDEL Voices newsletter: Voices from the Classroom.* Retrieved from http://www. ddelcec.org/DDEL_Newsletter.php

Noguera, P.A. (2002). Beyond size: The challenge of high school reform. *Educational Leadership,* 59(5), 60-63.

Weinberg, L.A., Zetlin, A., and Shea, N.M. (2009). Removing barriers to educating children in foster care through interagency collaboration: A seven county multiple-case study. *Child Welfare,* 88(4), 77-111.

Scherr, T.G. (2007). Education experiences of children in foster care: Meta-analyses of special education, retention and discipline rates. *School Psychology International*, 28(4), 419-436.

Shea, N., Weinberg, L., Zetlin, A. (2011). *Meeting the challenge: A preliminary report on the education performance of foster youth in three California counties.* Los Angeles, Mental Health Advocacy Services, Inc.

Zetlin, A., Weinberg, L., and Kimm, C. (2004). Improving educational outcomes for children in foster care: Interventions by an education liaison. *Journal of Education for Students Placed at Risk (JESPAR)*, 9(4), 421-429.

Zetlin, A.G., Weinberg, L.A., and Shea, N.M., (2006a). Seeing the whole picture: Views from diverse participants on barriers to educating foster youth. *Children and Schools*, 28(3), 165-173.

Zetlin, A.G., Weinberg, L.A., and Shea, N.M. (2006b). Improving educational prospects for youth in foster care: The educational liaison model. *Intervention in School and Clinic*, 41(5), 257-272.

Zetlin, A.G., Weinberg, L.A., and Shea, N.M., (2010). Caregivers, school liaisons, and agency advocates speak out about the educational needs of children and youths in foster care. *Social Work*, 55(3), 245-253.

In: Child Welfare
Editors: Alex Powell and Jenna Gray-Peterson

ISBN: 978-1-62257-826-9
© 2013 Nova Science Publishers, Inc.

Chapter 6

DEVELOPING A CHILD WELFARE AND CHILD PROTECTION SYSTEM IN CHINA: UNICEF SUPPORT TO THE GOVERNMENT OF CHINA

Lisa Ng Bow

ABSTRACT

China faces many complex new challenges in light of the current trends of rapid economic growth, urbanization, massive domestic migration, dislocation and separation of family members, changing family structures, increasing cost of basic social services, rising disparities, and increasing frequency of natural disasters. In this current context, children and their families are increasingly exposed to new social welfare and child protection risks, with poverty acting as a contributing factor to the risk of child protection violations. As it has become more difficult for the Chinese government to manage these risks and vulnerabilities through vertical social protection programs, China is beginning to shift from an issues-based approach to social welfare and child protection toward a more comprehensive, multisectoral child welfare and child protection system as the most effective way to address new challenges. This new system comprises a social welfare system that provides (a) universal benefits to support social protection and services for all children and their families, and within this, (b) a child protection system that targets the most vulnerable children.

UNICEF is supporting the Chinese government to strengthen its social welfare system for children at three basic levels: (a) at the upstream and national level, supporting the development of child-sensitive national social protection, social assistance and child protection policies, laws, and frameworks; (b) at the intermediate or provincial level, developing strategies, mechanisms, and plans that facilitate the implementation of national child welfare and child protection laws and policies; and (c) at the community level, piloting and demonstrating effective, affordable, and sustainable intersectoral child welfare and child protection packages and models within diverse local settings for possible government replication (this component also feeds into policy development).

Within this social welfare framework, UNICEF is supporting China to move toward the establishment of a child protection system; this involves policy and legal reforms aimed at a strengthening a systems approach to child protection which is integrally linked with the social welfare and justice systems. Support is also being provided to demonstrate and develop community-based child protection service models that prevent and respond to violence, abuse, exploitation, and neglect.

Keywords: China, UNICEF, Child welfare, Child protection, Social work, Social welfare, Social protection, Children without caregivers, Orphans, Abandoned children, Children with disabilities, Children living in poverty, Street children, Children in conflict with the law, Trafficked children, Migrant children, Left-behind children

I. Current Social Economic Context and Trends in China: Implications for Children

Since initiating economic reforms in the late 1970s, China has achieved remarkable economic growth and advances in poverty reduction. Based on the international poverty line of US$1.25 a day, the proportion of China's population living in income poverty declined from 81.6% in 1981 to 10.4% in 2005 (Chen and Ravallion, 2008). Based on China's national poverty line of 1,196 RMB per capita, the country's rural poor population dropped dramatically from 250 million in 1978 to about 36 million in 2009 (Ministry of Foreign Affairs and UN-China, 2010).

China's progress in terms of poverty alleviation and efforts to bolster social protection has, in turn, led to substantial improvements in the quality of life for the vast majority of the population.

These developments have also resulted in significant progress in relation to the survival, development, and protection of children. Between 1991 and 2009, the under-five mortality rate declined from 61 to 17 per 1,000 live births (MOH, 2009). From 1990 to 2005, the prevalence of underweight among children under five decreased from 19% to 7% (China Center for Disease Control, 2005). Nationally, the net enrolment rate for primary education reached 99.4% in 2009 (NBS, 2010), while the gross enrolment rate for junior secondary education rose from 67% in 1991 to 98.5% in 2008 (MOE, 2009).

Alongside these achievements, however, China faces many new challenges in the current development context. Despite the national economic boom that has occurred over the past three decades, the absolute number of people living in income poverty across the country - 135.4 million people - remains extremely high and poverty in many areas remains deeply entrenched. Given current trends, including continued rapid economic growth, increasing inequalities among regions and population groups, accelerated urbanization, massive internal migration, frequent dislocation and separation of family members, and the greater frequency of natural disasters, the Chinese government faces a complex set of new challenges.

In the context of these trends, children and their families, especially the poorest and most disadvantaged, are increasingly exposed to social welfare and child protection risks. Moreover, almost a fifth of the rural population remains highly vulnerable to falling into poverty due to income shocks, loss of employment, illness or accidents, natural disasters, and other adverse economic and social conditions (World Bank, 2009).

As a result, it has become increasingly difficult to ensure that all children throughout the country in need of support, especially those most vulnerable to violence, abuse, exploitation and neglect, are able to benefit from the existing child welfare and child protection programs.

Increasing Burden of Health Care and Education Costs on Families

While China's economic reforms have lifted over 200 million people out of poverty, economic restructuring and the transition to a market economy have also generated some negative outcomes. With the dismantling of the commune system and publicly financed social welfare provisions and the subsequent marketization and introduction of user fees for social services, the affordability of and access to basic social services have declined substantially (World Bank, 2009). In addition, financial responsibilities for the provision of public social services have been decentralized from central level to lower administrative levels. This has meant that social services provision has become highly dependent on the fiscal capacity of local governments. Local fiscal capacity is, in turn, strongly correlated with the level of economic development of a particular province or administrative area. While mandated to provide social services to the local population, many poorer provinces, counties, and villages lack the resources to do so (Dollar, 2007). Moreover, field research has indicated that the general decline in public goods and services provision over the past few decades is not only a result of fiscal decentralization, but also of weak accountability frameworks and incentive structures at the village level that have led public officials to prioritize investment in economic growth over social public goods and services (Tsai, 2007).

Thus, families living below or near the poverty line continue to struggle to pay for the rising costs of health care services and education, and consequently, some are forced to limit or sometimes forego these services. A World Bank study estimated that between 1980 and 2004, out-of-pocket household expenditure on health care increased 40-fold (World Bank, 2006). A different study found that educational expenses for a year of primary school and a year of secondary school constituted 40% and 70%, respectively, of the official poverty line (World Bank, 2009). Respondents from yet another survey in 2006 indicated that the main causes for poverty were rising health expenditure, the cost of children's education, and insufficient agricultural income (China Development Research Foundation, 2007).

Central-level fiscal transfers provide a basic level of support to provincial and local governments, and total government expenditure on education and health has increased in recent years. Following the launch of health sector reforms in 2009, government health expenditure rose to 1.4% of GDP and health insurance coverage increased significantly (MOH, 2010). In 2009, total government expenditure on education was 3.6% of GDP (MOE, 2010). However, there are concerns that these new investments in health and education will not translate into reduced disparities at the subnational level. The overwhelming burden of financing social services falls on provincial and lower level governments, and the subnational administration of social services is prone to operational inefficiencies (Brixi et al., 2011). Tsai's (2007) findings on weak accountability and distorted incentive frameworks at village level also point to additional barriers to the equitable provision of public social services. This has resulted in negative outcomes and increased vulnerability for children and their families, especially in poor counties.

Massive Rural-to-Urban Migration

In 2009, an estimated 211 million migrants in China moved from mainly rural areas to cities (National Population and Family Planning Commission, 2010). Among this "floating population", there were approximately 27.25 million children who had migrated to the cities with their parents in 2008 (NBS, 2008). In addition, about 55 million children were left behind in rural areas by one or both migrating parents (Office of Migrant Workers and ACWF, 2008).

Under the household registration system in China, social benefits and access to services are tied to a person's urban or rural household registration or *hukou*.[1] Benefits allowed under rural social assistance and social protection programs are not portable across provincial and municipal borders. Migrants with a rural *hukou* living in urban areas are often only provided with temporary urban residence status, and therefore they do not enjoy the same rights, social services, and protection as registered urban populations. To access public services or social protection, migrants need to return to their place of official rural *hukou* residence, which clearly is not practical. As a result, in terms of access to public health care and public schools in the cities where they live, migrant children do not have the same rights as their urban counterparts. This has resulted in higher rates of mortality and morbidity (such as vaccine-preventable diseases) among migrant children, which in turn, may threaten the health of urban residents. Similarly, the parents of migrant children do not benefit equally from social services and social protection programs, such as unemployment insurance and a pension. This leaves migrant families extremely vulnerable and considerably disadvantaged.

For the children left in rural areas, the loss of direct parental care and protection can have long-term negative effects on their physical, educational, and psychological development and well-being. Substitute caregivers, often illiterate grandparents, frequently do not have up-to-date knowledge on parenting or child-rearing skills and are unable to adequately supervise the health, nutrition, education, care, and protection of these children (Duan, 2005).[2] Children left in rural areas by migrating parents also tend to spend an increasing amount of time on family agricultural work in order to fill the labor gap left by migrating parents; this leaves less time for school and other activities. While not all left-behind children are vulnerable, the lack of sufficient adult supervision raises serious child protection concerns. In recent years, there have been increasing reports of criminal networks and trafficking agents targeting both left-behind children and migrant children, whose parents are often unable to provide adequate supervision as they struggle to earn a living.

In addition, with the easing of restrictions on migration, large population movements, and more developed transportation routes, children in general are more exposed to the risk of trafficking as well as to HIV/AIDS. Young, poor, or socially isolated segments of the rural population, who often do not have adequate knowledge, life skills, or negotiating power to protect themselves, are also at a higher risk of exploitation and abuse, such as trafficking for child labor, sexual exploitation, illegal marriages, and various forms of violence.

With the total migrant population anticipated to rise to 350 million by 2050 (NPFPC, 2010), a well-developed and comprehensive social welfare and child protection system that includes specific new elements for urban migrants is critical to ensuring universal and equitable access to social services, prevention services and protection for all children.

---

[1] The government *hukou* system, introduced in 1958 to regulate urbanization, requires household members to register as legal residents with their local public security offices. In 1984, rural laborers were permitted to move to the cities to seek jobs, and this led to a massive migration to more economically developed urban areas.

[2] A UNICEF project baseline study showed that more than 50% of children left in rural areas grow up with a single parent and 47% are entrusted to the care of grandparents, other relatives, or, in some cases, their siblings. About 40% of all left-behind children below the age of 5 years live with their grandparents.

Demographic Shifts

The demographic profile of China is changing. Following the introduction of China's family planning policy in 1979 (known as the "One Child Policy") and changing social attitudes on family size, the total fertility rate declined from about 5 to 1.77 births per woman between 1970 and 2010 (UNFPA, 2010). With the declining number of births and an increasing life span in China, the country has an aging population. Without an adequate social security system, younger generations are faced with increasing pressure to financially support both their parents and grandparents in old age.

At the same time, within the Chinese context of declining total fertility rates, the increased availability of affordable sex-selection technology, and son preference, the number of boys born compared to girls has also risen. While the global demographic norm for the sex ratio at birth ranges between 103 and 107 male births to every 100 female births, China's sex ratio at birth increased from a relatively normal rate of 108.5 male births to every 100 female births in 1982 to 120.5 male births to every 100 female births in 2005 (NBS, 2005, 2007). There are currently 23.77 million more males than females under the age of 19 in China (Xinhua, 2011). By 2020, it is estimated that males of this age will outnumber their female counterparts by 30 to 40 million (The Economist, 2010).

This large sex imbalance has social implications. Experts suggest that the rising violence and crime rates in the past decade are associated with the increasing number of men unable to marry, and moreover, they anticipate that the overall level of crime and societal violence will be further exacerbated in the coming decades as those born under the family planning policies initiated in 1979 reach marrying age (Edlund et al., 2009). Sexual violence and exploitation in particular are anticipated to rise. A 2005 UNICEF-supported Peking University survey carried out in six provinces and municipalities found the existing prevalence rate of sexual violence to be almost 29% for girls before the age of 16 and 22% for boys (Peking University, 2005). The sex ratio imbalance is already presumed to be a contributing factor in the rising incidence of abductions and trafficking of young women and girls for forced early marriages, prostitution, and sexual exploitation (Waldmeir, 2011).

In the context of Chinese social norms and attitudes, lower total fertility rates have been accompanied by other social consequences. In China, there is tradition of son preference, and this has contributed to the increased trafficking in infant boys for illegal adoption. Lower fertility rates combined with negative social attitudes about children with disabilities and the lack of support services for families with disabled children are believed to be linked to the disproportionately high number of children with disabilities being abandoned in child welfare institutions (CWIs). In 2008, research undertaken with families and CWIs in major cities across China found that over 90% of children living in CWIs were children with disabilities (Shang et al., 2010).

Rising Inequalities

Finally, in the context of rapid growth, China has experienced rising income and human development disparities among different geographical regions of the country and population groups, especially between western, remote, or rural regions and urban areas and between migrating and resident populations. Infant and child mortality in western regions is almost 2.7

times higher than in eastern regions and 2.4 times higher in rural areas compared to urban areas (UNICEF, 2009). More dramatically, the highest provincial under-five mortality rate is eight times the lowest. There are lower rates of access to public health care and education among migrant children. Based on a 2004 survey, only 37% of migrant children received full vaccination coverage. A study on maternal mortality in Ningbo, Zhejiang Province found an estimated maternal mortality ratio of 128 per 100,000 live births for migrant women in these areas compared to 9.5 among women who were permanent residents (China Health Economics Institute, 2006).

The Gini coefficient (a measure of a country's income inequality) in China rose from 0.27 in 1984 to about 0.44 in 2006, reflecting the increasingly uneven development across the country (Chen et al., 2010). Higher Gini coefficients are often associated with increases in social instability. As China continues on its path of rapid economic growth, it will be important to develop a more comprehensive child welfare and social protection system to ensure that the needs of different population groups are met and their vulnerabilities effectively addressed. This will help guard against the further widening of disparities and support social stability.

II. UNICEF's Approach to a Comprehensive Child Welfare and Protection System

A. Supporting a Systems-based Approach to Child Welfare

Globally, social welfare systems not only aim to reduce income poverty but also to address issues of risk, vulnerability, and social exclusion. The most effective social welfare policies are those that provide universal support as well as specific policies and support for the most vulnerable. Interventions targeting the risks associated with vulnerable groups, such as the poor, elderly, disabled persons, unemployed, children, and families, are therefore one way of achieving universal access to assistance and social protection. Thus, UNICEF's approach to child welfare and child protection in China and across the world has been to support government efforts to promote universal benefits and to strengthen integrated policies and services in order to prevent child protection problems and to respond to the specific needs of children and families who are at risk of significant harm. Significant harm refers to harm to a child causing a long-term or lifelong negative impact.

While low-income countries tend to focus on developing a minimum package of child welfare and protection services with supporting policies and capacities, middle-income countries often work on reforming existing social and legal systems, with attention focused on improving multisectoral coordination, social protection, the rule of law, and gender equality (UNICEF, 2008). As a middle-income country that is undergoing rapid economic development and that has already established social assistance and protection programs, China is well positioned to strengthen its national child welfare and child protection system. Indeed, China is keen to develop a child welfare system that corresponds to its level of economic development. In recent years, the Chinese government has taken the initial steps toward developing a comprehensive child welfare and child protection system, one which has begun to build universal benefits alongside targeted interventions for vulnerable groups.

B. Child Protection as Part of the Broader Social Welfare System

The child protection system is an essential part of the larger national social welfare system for children. While social welfare systems are different in every country and are best determined by the countries themselves according to local conditions, they often encompass a wide range of policies, including social assistance, social insurance, social services, livelihood and employment policy, and child protection and family support policies. In light of the complex development challenges faced by China, the government would greatly benefit from developing a comprehensive child protection system as part of the country's overall social welfare system.

C. Rationale for UNICEF's Systems-based Approach to Child Protection

Globally, the aim of UNICEF's child protection work is to help develop a protective environment where girls and boys are free from violence, abuse, exploitation, and unnecessary separation from family. To promote this aim, UNICEF supports the development of laws, services, behaviors, and practices designed to minimize children's vulnerability, address known risk factors, and strengthen children's personal resilience (UNICEF, 2008).

UNICEF works closely with governments across the world to achieve this goal in accordance with international child rights frameworks, norms, and standards. Article 19 of the Convention on the Rights of the Child, which reflects government obligations in relation to child protection, states:

> "**State** parties shall take all appropriate legislative, administrative, social and educational measures to protect the child from all forms of physical or mental violence, injury or abuse, neglect and negligent treatment, maltreatment or exploitation, including sexual abuse, while in the care of parent(s), legal guardian(s) or any other **person who has the care of the child**" (United Nations, 1989).

Many countries tend to approach child protection through interventions addressing specific categories of children, such as street children, trafficked children, and orphaned children. In parallel, government agencies often carry out interventions focused on a single child protection issue without sufficient collaboration with other government sectors. This occurs for various reasons, including vertically organized institutional arrangements, donor or government resources directed toward one category of vulnerable children, and new initiatives emerging from sudden media attention on a specific issue. The resulting gap in terms of the coverage of child protection areas and the necessary linkages between them results in a less strategic and less efficient and effective use of resources for child protection (UNICEF, 2008).

Most children in need of protection have multiple vulnerabilities and face various risks at the same time or over a period of time; therefore, they cannot all be categorized within one vulnerable group or another. For example, unsupervised children left behind in poor rural areas by migrating parents are more vulnerable to trafficking and may be trafficked into child labor or sold for illegal adoption. A child physically abused by her family may run away from home and become a child living on the streets; under traditional single-issue interventions, authorities might return the street child to her abusive family without addressing the underlying issue of abuse in the family or facilitating the provision of essential services or support. Ultimately, the specific needs of the individual child, which are likely to be multifaceted, must be met. Responding to these needs and preventing a broad range of vulnerabilities, rather than providing narrow services associated with one category of abuse or exploitation, should be the focus of child protection services.

The prevention and response services needed by an abused child should involve cooperation between community workers spread across many different sectors, such as health care workers and teachers to report suspected cases of child abuse, community-based social workers to investigate cases and provide monitoring and case management, and support families to change abusive behaviors and identify alternative care as needed. Thus, fragmented child protection responses may respond to one issue, but in most child protection cases, coordination among many sectors is necessary to meet the multidimensional needs of the child in a sustainable, meaningful way.

The interlinked nature of child protection issues underscores the need for a comprehensive, integrated child protection system that addresses the different vulnerabilities of children. International experiences and lessons have shown that a systems-based approach to child protection in which laws, social services, behaviors, and practices work together to reduce children's vulnerability and risk factors is the most effective way to prevent and respond to the interrelated risk factors and vulnerabilities associated with violence, abuse, exploitation, and neglect.

D. Key Components of a Child Protection System (UNICEF EAPRO, 2009)

Worldwide, UNICEF defines a child protection system as a set of laws, policies, regulations, and services needed across all social sectors to support prevention and responses to protection-related risks and safeguard children against all forms of abuse, exploitation, violence, and neglect. The social sectors that have particularly important roles to play are social welfare, education, health, security, and justice. Child protection systems should be readily accessible, including during emergencies and conflicts.

An effective child protection system consists of three key components—a legal and regulatory system, a social welfare system, and a social behavior change component—which work together to reduce children's vulnerability.

The *legal and regulatory framework* provides the laws and policies that set out the legal basis for preventing and responding to child violence, abuse, exploitation, and neglect. Effective enforcement mechanisms also form a key part of this component, helping to ensure that laws and policies are followed and regulated. The justice sector is also essential in strengthening accountability and the rule of law and denying impunity for violations.

The *social welfare system* provides a range of family support and child protection services operationalized at community level that help to prevent and respond to violence, abuse, exploitation, and neglect involving children. This system encompasses prevention services that help to reduce social exclusion, risk, and vulnerability. It also provides identification, investigation, referral, and response services; family support services; recovery and reintegration services; and counseling and psychosocial support mechanisms. These services need to be readily accessible at the community level, sufficiently financed, and adequately staffed by qualified social workers.

The *social behavior change component* aims to promote attitudes, beliefs, values, and behaviors that support children's well-being and protection. This involves raising public awareness of the social and cultural behaviors, norms, and practices that can have a negative or positive impact on a child's development. This is commonly done through national and provincial public awareness campaigns, as well as through local community and family education services. Such services are critical to reinforcing good behavioral norms (e.g., positive parenting practices or zero tolerance of corporal punishment) within different settings (e.g., households, schools, institutions).

These three components also require meaningful interaction. Laws and policy frameworks delineate what is formally permitted by governments, which then guides and influences social behavior and norms. Conversely, prevailing cultural beliefs and social norms influence what is actually practiced at the local level and the extent to which child protection laws and policies are implemented. For example, if child abuse is widely tolerated as a socially acceptable practice, a law prohibiting child abuse may have limited effect and behavior change communication and advocacy may be needed to alter social and cultural attitudes in order to reduce child abuse.

Similarly, although child protection laws and policies may outline the framework for a child protection system and the social services to be provided, if services are not available to support implementation (e.g., due to the lack of well-trained social workers or a lack of funding for community-level services) or if the justice system does not respond effectively to enforce the law or guard against impunity, then child protection initiatives will be much less effective. By the same token, if social services are widely available but community uptake is low due to a lack of awareness of the services, to poor quality services, or to prevailing negative attitudes of service providers, then child protection interventions will not be successful, thus resulting in negative outcomes for children. Therefore, all three components are vital to an effective children protection system.

III. The Existing Child Welfare and Child Protection System in China

In China, as in many parts of the world, child welfare and protection were traditionally considered to be family matters to be addressed within the private domain. Thus, the Chinese government initially adopted a traditional issues-based approach to child welfare and child protection, focusing primarily on protecting and supporting children without parental care, especially street children, abandoned children, and orphans. As new developments and child protection challenges emerged, the government introduced various new social assistance schemes, and these schemes have had a positive impact on the lives of poor and vulnerable children. However, the social and economic costs of inadequate child protection systems and the impact of violence against children and the abuse, exploitation, and neglect of children on both the children themselves and on society are gradually being recognized. These costs range from poor educational achievement and human capacity loss to rising public sector expenditures on medical treatment as a result of child injuries and increased criminality stemming from childhood violence and abuse. Thus, the protection of children is being increasingly understood as a government responsibility and a public policy issue.

The Chinese government is also starting to recognize the limitations of narrow social assistance schemes vertical government structures, and programs targeting specific categories of children in addressing child welfare and protection problems. It is therefore beginning to move toward a more integrated approach to addressing these issues. This approach includes supporting interventions to reduce poverty and providing basic social services on a more universal basis, as well as providing an increasingly multisectoral approach to preventing and responding to children at risk of significant harm from violence, abuse, exploitation, and neglect (Di Martino, Shi, and Chen, 2010).

The effectiveness and benefits of this comprehensive approach were evidenced in UNICEF-supported child welfare demonstration pilots for children affected by HIV/AIDS and children in need of special protection.

Public social service provision in these pilots prioritized first and foremost children's access to basic essential services, such as health care, education, and social protection, as something that all children need. However, given their special vulnerability, children affected by HIV/AIDS and children in need of special protection also require access to specialized child protection services to prevent stigma, discrimination, violence, abuse, and exploitation.

The sections below discuss the current social welfare system and highlight the child protection components within it.

A. Social Welfare and Child Protection Policy Frameworks

In light of the development challenges described in Part I, China has accelerated its efforts in relation to poverty alleviation and social economic development and has been strengthening its social welfare and protection system, particularly over the past decade.

National Development and Social Welfare Policy Frameworks

Over the past 15 years, the Chinese government has adopted several major poverty reduction strategies and policies for rural areas that have significantly contributed to reducing the poverty risks for vulnerable populations. These measures have included China's Western Region Development Strategy (2000), area-based poverty programs (2001), and policies supporting farmers, such as the elimination of agricultural taxes in 2006 and the provision of agricultural subsidies and training for farmers in 2004 (World Bank, 2009).

In 2004, in response to rising inequalities and social tensions, China adopted the Resolution on Major Issues Regarding the Building of a Harmonious Socialist Society. This resolution called for more balanced, equitable growth; greater attention to social equity and justice; and increased emphasis on resolving social conflicts underpinned by improved public administration and social welfare services. The goal of developing a harmonious society (*he xie she hui*) continues to guide social economic policies and policy implementation in China today.

In 2011, the Government finalized its 12th National Five-Year Plan for Social and Economic Development (2011–2015). This plan, which outlines a shift in strategy from export-oriented economic growth toward domestic demand-driven growth, reflects a parallel need to increase the incomes of poor families and to strengthen social security and protection systems in order to encourage sustainable domestic consumption. China also issued its Ten-year Poverty Reduction Strategy (2011-2020) in 2011; this includes measures to strengthen child-sensitive investments and policies and reflects the key dimensions of the child poverty issue.

International Treaties Related to Children

China has ratified many international treaties and rights instruments to support the protection and promotion of the well-being of children in China. These instruments have presented China with guiding frameworks, international standards, and norms that have contributed to the development of domestic child welfare and protection policies, laws, and national plans of action.

As an early signatory to the 1989 United Nations Convention on the Rights of the Child (CRC), the Chinese government in 1992 pledged to meet its commitment to respect, promote, and fulfill the social, educational, economic, cultural, civil, and political rights of children. China also ratified the two optional protocols of the CRC—the Optional Protocol on the Involvement of Children in Armed Conflict in 2008 and the Optional Protocol on the Sale of Children, Child Prostitution and Child Pornography in 2002— and two other important treaties: the Convention on the Elimination of All Forms of Discrimination against Women in 1981 and the ILO Convention on the Worst Forms of Child Labor in 2002.

To strengthen antitrafficking measures across countries, China acceded to the UN Protocol to Prevent, Suppress and Punish Trafficking in Persons, Especially Women and Children (known as the Palermo Protocol) in 2010, ratified the Hague Convention on the Protection of Children and Cooperation in Respect of Intercountry Adoption in 2005, and signed two bilateral memorandums of understanding (MOUs), one with Myanmar (in 2009) and one with Vietnam (in 2010), to increase cooperation in preventing and responding to human trafficking. China is now in the process of discussing antitrafficking MOUs with other bordering countries.

National Child Welfare and Child Protection Policy Frameworks

China has developed several national plans of action (NPAs) to mobilize and coordinate the implementation of child welfare and protection measures across sectors. Foremost is China's National Plan of Action for Children's Development, which provides the main policy framework for implementing the CRC. In mid-2011, China formally released its new NPA for 2011-2020. Importantly, for the first time, the new NPA has child welfare as one of its five main pillars. This has set the stage for building a more comprehensive, systemic approach to child welfare work in the future, an approach aimed at developing more universal community-based, family-focused child welfare services. This NPA also identified child protection as another major pillar, highlighting the need to strengthen the protection of children at risk and to establish a community-based system to report, identify, and respond to violence against children (NPA for Children's Development, 2011)[3]

China is also in process of developing several key child-welfare-specific policy frameworks, including the 12th National Plan of Action for Child Welfare (2011-2015), the

---

[3] The children at risk and in need of protection include abandoned and orphaned children; street children; children affected by natural disasters, migration, and HIV/AIDS; and children whose parents are serving prison sentences.

Child Welfare Act, and the Five-year National Plan on the Development of Social Work for Children.

The Law on the Protection of Minors is one of the main laws governing child protection in China. The Chinese government expanded protection for children under a 2006 revision of this law by further delineating the responsibilities of families, schools, and government in relation to child and judicial protection.

With regard to the child protection categories of trafficking, street children, and migrant children, China has been developing multisectoral frameworks to improve coordination. With regard to antitrafficking work, China is in the process of developing its second National Plan of Action on Combating Trafficking in Women and Children (2013-2017) to better coordinate national efforts. The first trafficking NPA (2008-2012) helped to improve antitrafficking coordination and security mechanisms, clarify the different responsibilities of relevant government departments, and establish longer term antitrafficking mechanisms focused on prevention, assistance, and rehabilitation. Related to this, the government also revised the national Penal Code, outlining harsher penalties for trafficking criminals.

To better protect children living on the street, the State Council released the Opinion on Strengthening the Protection and Assistance to Street Children in August 2011, which authorized the establishment of a national interministerial working mechanism to protect street children. This document underscored the need to strengthen prevention and reintegration measures, family support, and access to formal or nonformal education for street children. It also allows courts to remove the custodial rights of parents or legal guardians who allow their children to beg or steal on the streets.

With respect to children affected by migration, the State Council issued an opinion in 2006 which called on the government to reduce discrimination against migrant children and improve their right to education and to improve interministerial coordination to support left-behind children (State Council, 2006). Since then, a number of municipal governments have introduced policies to improve access to compulsory education for migrant children (Shang and Wang, 2011).

For children without parental care, China has developed several government policies on adoption and on family-like, kinship, and foster care for children without caregivers. These policies include the 1992 Adoption Law, guiding frameworks for domestic and international adoptions, and policies managing family-like foster care.

Regulations establishing parameters for the institutional care of children without caregivers have also been issued; among other items, the basic requirements for food, care, rehabilitation services for children with disabilities, psychosocial support, education, and physical facilities were outlined (Shang and Wang, 2011).

These new child welfare and multisectoral child protection frameworks are significant in that they provide the broad policy frameworks and the initial basis for a systems approach. However, the next set of challenges will include implementing these frameworks at provincial and lower level and departing from sectoral activities aggregated around traditional child protection issues toward more deeply integrated policies, and a continuum of services that benefits from active intersectoral engagement and a primary focus on prevention of risk and vulnerability.

B. Social Assistance Schemes, Social Insurance, Fee Waivers, and Services

In addition to laws and policy frameworks, China has introduced a wide range of social assistance schemes, social insurance, fee waivers, and child welfare and protection services for vulnerable groups. These measures have improved the social and economic security of families, providing a first line of protection for children. As a result, the child welfare and protection system has been strengthened. Other developments include substantial improvements in child nutrition, universal access to 9 years of compulsory education, and improved access to basic public health care services (UNICEF-China, 2010).

Social Assistance Schemes

The various social assistance schemes that have been adopted in China have helped to assist the poorest segments of the population to have the basic minimum living standards, and defend against further impoverishment. The *Tekun* scheme provides subsistence living assistance to extremely poor families living under the poverty line in rural areas. Recipients often have no means of supporting themselves due to illness, disability, injury, or disasters. Under the *Wubao* scheme (or five guarantees program), very poor households receive five basic items: food, clothing, housing, medical care, and funeral costs. This scheme, which is financed by local governments, serves three segments of the poor and vulnerable population—the elderly, people with disabilities, and children under 16—if they are unable to work, have no means of earning an income, and have no other form of support; this includes orphans and poor children with disabilities (Shang and Wang, 2011).

One of the most important and far reaching forms of social assistance is the *dibao* scheme. The urban *dibao* scheme (or minimum subsistence allowance program), with eligibility based on household per capita income, was set up in 1999 to support poor urban residents. A parallel rural *dibao* scheme was initiated in 2007, expanding this basic subsistence allowance nationally to rural residents. By the end of 2010, the *dibao* scheme was reported to have benefitted more than 75 million people: 23 million urban residents and over 52 million rural residents (Shang and Wang, 2011). This program, supported by local and central level funding, has helped to improve basic child nutrition and the uptake of health and education services by the poorest people in society.

The Medical Financial Assistance (MFA) scheme was initiated in rural areas in 2003 and in urban areas in 2005, and aims to offset the heavy financial burden of health care costs for poor households. This scheme, administered by the Ministry of Civil Affairs (MCA), provides support to cover health insurance premiums and copayments for impoverished households, as well as some out-of-pocket medical expenses for poor uninsured households. By 2007, the scheme had been established in all rural counties and 86% of cities; however, problems have been identified with regard to the targeting of beneficiaries (World Bank, 2009).

China, as a disaster-prone country, provides disaster relief assistance to affected populations, usually through a central fund providing cash transfers, food, clothing, reconstruction, and medical care. The Chinese government has increased disaster assistance in recent years, from 5.1 billion RMB in 2004 to 11.34 billion RMB in 2010 (MCA, 2009/2010). The scale of assistance varies with the severity of the disaster. After the devastating 2008 Wenchuan earthquake, for example, China provided almost 61 billion RMB to assist those affected, including a 600 RMB monthly subsidy for each child orphaned after the earthquake (World Bank, 2009).

China has also developed targeted social assistance programs for specific vulnerable groups, including children affected by HIV/AIDS and orphans. In 2003, China's introduced the "Four Frees and One Care" HIV/AIDS policy, which supports the provision of free prevention of mother-to-child transmission services and antiretroviral treatment as well as living support and education for children orphaned by AIDS. The pilot work of UNICEF and the MCA supported the implementation of this policy and produced four demonstration models of community-based care for children affected by AIDS. The care given since 2004 to orphans who have lost both parents was extended to all children affected by AIDS in 2009 following the issuance of China's 2009 Opinion on Enhanced Efforts in Welfare Protection for Children Affected by AIDS.

In October 2010, the State Council issued an important new policy in its Opinion on Strengthening Social Protection for Orphans, outlining government provisions to ensure a basic standard of living for orphans, as advocated through the joint MCA-UNICEF child welfare demonstration pilots. This policy states that all orphans should receive a monthly cash transfer: 1,000 RMB for orphans raised in institutional care and 600 RMB for orphans raised by kin or in foster care;[4] the latter is significant in that the government, for the first time, is providing a subsidy for care by kin and for foster care. The central government also allocated 2.5 billion RMB (about US$367 million) to provincial departments to support the implementation of this policy.

Social Insurance

Given the increasing vulnerability of families and children to poverty due to various shocks, China has introduced different social insurance schemes in rural and urban areas, and these have helped to improve social protection for families and the well-being of children.

Rural areas. The new Rural Cooperative Medical Scheme (RCMS), initially developed in the 1960s but then dismantled during the economic reform period, was relaunched in 2003. The RCMS is a major voluntary health insurance scheme for the rural population which is financed by central and local governments and individual contributions. The scheme aims to provide universal health insurance coverage in rural areas, and in 2009, it covered over 94% of the rural population (NBS, 2010). However, since the benefits mainly cover catastrophic illnesses and in-patient medical services and offer relatively low reimbursement rates, estimated at around 44% in 2008 (WHO, 2009), out-of-pocket costs remain prohibitively high, especially for the poor. Coverage and benefits are improving as funding of the scheme grows, but many poor households continue to forego certain basic health services due to the high out-of-pocket costs. In addition, rural families who migrate to cities for work cannot benefit from the RCMS.

The Basic Rural Pension Scheme, which was introduced in the late 1990s, covers rural residents between 20 and 60 years of age and is funded by individual contributions with some government support. Pension benefits are provided after participants reach the age of 60.

---

[4] Central-level funds are allocated to Chinese provinces by region, with the eastern Chinese provinces receiving 180 RMB per month per child; central Chinese provinces 270 RMB per month per child; and Western Chinese provinces 360 RMB per month per child. While the total central-level contribution is significant, provincial- and county-level authorities still need to provide supplementary funding to meet the minimum living standard criteria outlined, and this poses difficulties for poorer counties.

However, actual coverage under this pension scheme remains low, with only about 72.8 million rural residents qualifying for the basic pension in 2009, and no system exists to allow the portability of benefits for internal migrants (World Bank, 2009).

Urban areas. In urban areas, the Chinese government has strengthened social security by providing five types of protection under its Social Insurance Fund: basic medical insurance, unemployment insurance, work injury insurance, maternity insurance, and a pension.

China introduced basic medical insurance (BMI) in 1998 in order to provide health insurance coverage for urban workers in the formal sector. In 2009, this insurance scheme covered over 219 million workers and about 55 million retirees. Building on the BMI, the government introduced Urban Resident Basic Medical Insurance (URBMI) in 2007, offering voluntary basic health insurance for the unemployed urban population, including students and children not covered by the BMI. In 2009, the URBMI covered more than 182 million people (NBS, 2010). Like the RCMS, these two schemes are financed by central government, local funds, and individual contributions.

Unemployment insurance was made more widely available in 1999 as large numbers of workers in state-owned enterprises were being laid off due to economic restructuring. Under certain criteria, this scheme provides a maximum of 2 years of unemployment allowance, with medical subsidies in cases of illness. By 2009, this scheme covered over 127 million urban enterprise employees and government workers.

Work injury insurance, which is funded by employers, insures enterprise and business employees against medical expenses for work-related injuries and diseases. Benefits provide allowances for disability and injury and nursing fees, but these vary according to the sector and the level of occupational hazard. Recently, the government expanded coverage to rural migrant workers employed in high-risk jobs such as construction. In 2009, almost 149 million workers participated in this scheme.

Maternity insurance provides female enterprise employees and female urban workers in government agencies and other public organizations with 90 days of paid maternity leave and covers the cost of medical expenses during pregnancy. There were 108.75 million workers covered by maternity insurance in 2009.

The social insurance fund also supports the Basic Urban Pension scheme; in 2009, this scheme covered nearly 235.5 million people.

Fee Waivers or Fee Reductions

Health care services. China's 1995 Law on Maternal and Infant Health formally assigned the state with the responsibility to ensure that women and infants receive basic maternal and child health care services. In support of primary health care, the government supports the basic management of childhood diseases through the provision of health care services supporting disease prevention in children under five. In 2001, the State Council introduced Implementation Rules for the Maternal and Infant Health Law; these rules provide more practical guidance on implementing the law and outline the various responsibilities of different government and medical institutions for maternal and child health services. Neither law, however, requires services to be provided free of charge.

However, the government has since outlined various fee waivers, fee reductions, subsidies, and free services to promote access to maternal and child health care services, including immunization, maternal supplements, and maternal and newborn screening. Under the National Plan of Action on the Expanded Programme on Immunization (EPI) issued by the Ministry of Health (MOH) in 2007, China has supported universal access to vaccinations by waiving immunization service fees and has expanded the number of diseases covered under the EPI to 15. The government has also allocated 2,720 million RMB for vaccines, syringes, and health worker allowances to facilitate vaccinations in poor areas.

In 2000, China began to provide subsidies for poor rural women to deliver babies in hospital; this scheme was expanded to all rural counties in 2009. In addition, free folic acid supplements and breast and cervical cancer screenings for rural women were initiated in 2009. The government also introduced new measures for screening for diseases in newborns. In 2010, the MOH and the MCA issued an opinion to initiate work on increasing health care coverage and protection for rural children with serious diseases (Shang and Wang, 2011). Free treatment for certain communicable diseases (such as AIDS, tuberculosis, and schistosomiasis) has also been provided. To support children with intellectual disabilities, the MCA issued a policy statement in 2009 which focused on accelerating access to services for these children and set a target of reaching 5,000 children a year from 2009 to 2011. This policy was introduced in the context of the finding of a 2006 survey that 61% of children with disabilities never received the services intended for them.[5]

Education services. The 1998 Compulsory Education Law outlines the right of all children in China to receive 9 years of compulsory education: 6 years of primary school and 3 years of junior secondary education. In 2006, in an effort to increase universal access to 9 years of compulsory education, the government abolished tuition, textbook, and miscellaneous fees and provided boarding school subsistence for poor rural families; these benefits were extended to urban areas in 2007. Fiscal transfers from central to provincial and local governments help schools to offset the losses incurred as a result of the abolition of tuition and other fees, while county governments bear the cost of boarding subsidies.

More recently, in 2010, the State Council, in its Opinion on the Development of Preschool Education, outlined government plans to increase expenditure on early childhood development (ECD). The Chinese government will finance the construction of new preschool facilities, support private centers, improve training and benefits for teachers, and provide educational subsidies to rural areas. The government has also committed itself to making 1 year of preschool education universal by 2020. Over the past decade, the Ministry of Education (MOE) has piloted ECD initiatives in less developed rural areas, and these have demonstrated the tremendous benefits of ECD.

With regard to children with disabilities, a 1994 policy issued by the China Disabled Persons' Federation (CDPF) and the MOE formally established the right of children with disabilities to enter public schools. The Compulsory Education Law reinforces this right by emphasizing the responsibility of public schools to enroll children with disabilities. Subsequent policies have promoted the increased enrolment rate of disabled children into public schools. However, in terms of educational access, major gaps remain (Shang and Wang, 2011). With regard to other barriers to school enrolment, the MOH, the MOE, and the Ministry of Human Resources and Social Security jointly issued a circular in 2010 cancelling hepatitis B tests during health checks for school enrollment.

---

[5] The Second National Sample Survey on Disability conducted in 2006 by the China Disabled Persons' Federation found that 61% of children with disabilities never receive any of the services intended for those with disabilities (e.g., medical services, rehabilitation services, subsidies or exemptions for education fees, vocational training, employment placement and support, legal assistance, barrier-free facilities, and access to information and cultural services).

Child Welfare and Protection Services

The Chinese government's care and protection services for children originally focused on orphans, abandoned children, and street children, and thus existing institutional child protection structures reflect this focus. Across China, there are 303 CWIs and 800 social welfare institutions (SWIs) that provide alternative care for orphaned and abandoned children (Shang and Wang, 2011). According to the government, as of 2009, these institutions had supported over 115,000 children without parental care. There are also 1,400 relief centers, including 116 street children protection centers (SCPCs); as of 2009, these centers had provided temporary care and protection for about 145,000 street children. China has started to expand the services of CWIs and SWIs to include the facilitation of alternative care options, such as family-like foster care.

Diversifying Child Welfare and Child Protection Services

However, because the existing system of SWIs, CWIs, and SCPCs is unable to address the emerging complex and vast needs of all at-risk and vulnerable children, the Chinese government has begun to adopt a new strategy of diversifying the services provided by these institutions. The 2011-2020 NPA for Children's Development calls for (a) each urban and rural community to be staffed with at least one qualified child welfare professional and (b) one shelter for street children in each county and every city above prefecture level.

UNICEF has supported several CWIs and SCPCs in China[6] in diversifying their services in order to offer family support and community-based child welfare and protection services. The services these institutions provide to the children they serve include foster care, small-group family care for children under state care, rehabilitation services, parent education programs, social work support services, and outreach services to vulnerable children and their families.

Zhengzhou model for children living on the street. In 2001, the MCA, supported by UNICEF, began diversifying the child-friendly services available to children living on the streets in Zhengzhou City, Henan Province. The additional services offered by the Zhengzhou SCPC included outreach activities, street kiosks near bus terminals and train stations providing basic information and support, a drop-in center offering temporary shelter, rehabilitation services, referral services, a community-based residential center, facilitated foster care, informal education, vocational training for older children, and follow-up support for children returning home to their families.

The model has helped to provide temporary safe shelter to street children and to build their skills and capacity for independent living and decision making. It has also provided community-based family-like support, assistance with longer term living arrangements, and reintegration into mainstream society support.

The expansion to more comprehensive services has helped to significantly reduce the number of street children returning to live on the streets and has opened the doors to the provision of services for all vulnerable urban children – not just street children. The Chinese government has recognized the value of this pilot, now referred to as the Zhengzhou model, and has since replicated this model successfully in 15 cities across China.

---

[6] Diversified services were piloted in CWIs in Qingdao (Shandong), Yibin (Sichuan), and Urumqi (Xinjiang) and in SCPCs in Chengdu (Sichuan) and Panjin (Liaoning) with UNICEF support.

Child Protection Units. In 2006, child protection units (CPUs), piloted by the MCA and other partners with UNICEF support, developed a community-based mechanism focused on child protection. The CPUs aim to provide multisectoral prevention, identification, assessment, reporting, referral, and response services to children and families needing support, particularly in cases of violence against children and the abuse, exploitation, and neglect of children. A community-level database and monitoring system for vulnerable children has been set up to support the identification of at-risk, vulnerable families and children and case management by local social workers. To ensure collaboration from various sectors, CPUs involve the police, civil affairs workers, health workers, teachers, volunteers, parents, and children. The CPU model has helped to inform national strategies and local policies on developing a child protection system.

Child Friendly Spaces. Following the 2008 Wenchuan earthquake (Sichuan) and the 2010 Yushu earthquake (Qinghai), the National Working Committee for Children and Women (NWCCW) piloted a global UNICEF model called child friendly spaces (CFSs) and developed community-based CFSs in China. The CFSs established in Sichuan provided a safe community-based space for children to gather and engage in interactive group play activities aimed at helping children and their families to support each other and to obtain any other support needed to recover from the trauma of the earthquake. Other CFS services included registering vulnerable children and providing psychosocial support and counseling for children and their families.

Similar sites were set up in Yushu. To help children and families in post-disaster settings in the future, a Five-year Plan of Action on Social Work in Disaster Reconstruction and a Manual on Children and Social Work in Emergencies were developed. The CFS model and accompanying tools have improved government capacity to provide social work services in post-emergency settings.

In addition, the CFS model was adapted and replicated to provide community-based services to vulnerable migrant and left-behind children in rural areas. Services include registration, facilitated access to health and education services, family education for parents and caregivers, and psychosocial support. The CFS model, which is considered to be highly effective by government partners,[7] was included in the NPA for Children's Development (2011-2020) as a model for further replication.

Child welfare demonstration pilots. Child Welfare Demonstration Pilots, launched by the MCA in 2010 with UNICEF support, is a 6-year initiative supporting 120 villages within five provinces (Yunnan, Sichuan, Shanxi, Henan, and Xinjiang) with large numbers of vulnerable children. In these areas, many of the highly vulnerable are children affected by HIV/AIDS. The pilots are aimed at showing the value of a child welfare system approach by developing an essential package of child welfare services available to all children determining the cost of providing this service package and assessing its feasibility for wider replication.

With the critical support of community-level child welfare directors, the community centers identify and monitor vulnerable families and children and support their to access social services, including birth registration, family care and support, education, vocational training, health care, and income-generating activities.

---

[7] The 2010 midterm evaluation of CFSs in Sichuan by Peking University found that the CFSs established within quake-hit areas provide both a wide coverage of services and effective targeted services for vulnerable children and children with special needs which are "indisputably conducive for (the children's) sound development" and contribute to a rich culture of community.

Widening the Range of Social Work Service Providers, Including the Nonprofit Sector

Alongside these child welfare and child protection models, China is beginning to experiment with different models for government procurement of social work services through pilot "incubators" (*fu hua qi*). The models include incorporating the services of nongovernmental and voluntary groups into existing government social work service institutions, as well as government outsourcing social work services to registered nonprofit organizations. Experimentation with these models has been initiated in major cities such as Shanghai, Guangzhou, and Shenzhen. Given the immense need for child welfare and protection services at community level, the potential services and outreach provided by expanding the nonprofit sector could greatly assist in filling the current gap in social services. In the coming years, the government also plans to develop social welfare services in rural western and central areas through a human resource exchange program, in which a corps of qualified and experienced social workers from eastern coastal regions will train workers in these areas.

IV. REMAINING CHALLENGES FOR DEVELOPING A CHILD WELFARE AND PROTECTION SYSTEM

China has made progress in developing a more comprehensive child welfare and child protection system in the past three decades, reforming policy and legislative frameworks and expanding social welfare and child protection schemes and services to cover the most vulnerable families. China has achieved almost universal access to basic education and has greatly improved access to basic public health services. The new policy of providing cash transfers to orphans is also a positive step forward and opens the door to more universal approaches to social assistance for vulnerable children. However, some constraints remain.

Social Protection Coverage Has Expanded, but Average Benefits Are Low

While coverage in terms of social assistance, social insurance, fee waivers, and social services has expanded and increased considerably in both urban and rural areas in recent years, the average social benefits provided remain low in comparison to the poverty line and do not meet basic living standards for poor and vulnerable populations. According to a National Bureau of Statistics-World Bank study, in 2004, the village *dibao* scheme provided 65 RMB per person per year, representing a very small proportion of the 931 RMB per person per year poverty line (World Bank, 2009). Similarly, while the RCMS now provides almost universal rural health insurance coverage, RCMS benefits are often limited to catastrophic illnesses and in-patient medical services and reimbursement rates are low (NCMS Evaluation Task Force, 2006). Many people remain underinsured, face high out-of-pocket costs, and remain highly exposed to the risk of long-term poverty as a result of enormous health expenditure (UNICEF-China, 2008).

In addition, the coverage provided by the various health insurance programs in China varies over 60-fold between the RCMS and that available to workers in the state sector. Access to many publicly subsidized services, including antenatal care, basic and comprehensive emergency obstetric and newborn care, postnatal care, and infant screening, is below 50% in the rural areas of most western counties of China. Thus, poor families continue to struggle to meet basic living needs, secure adequate social protection, and obtain the essential services they require.

Implementation of Policy Frameworks at the Lower Level Remains Weak

At the policy level, the numerous legislative and policy frameworks for social welfare and child protection elaborated by the Chinese government provide a strong foundation for further developing a comprehensive child welfare system in China. However, for the reasons discussed in Part I, local implementation and enforcement—from provincial to village and community level—remain relatively weak. Weak upward and downward accountability mechanisms and distorted incentive structures at local level hamper the effectiveness of implementation. A 2006 citizen scorecard survey examining people's opinions and experiences with public service delivery demonstrated the value of citizen feedback for policy development and implementation and offers some promising possibilities (Brixi, 2009). In the absence of an effective coordination body and stronger accountability, monitoring, and enforcement mechanisms, the implementation of a system-based approach at various administrative levels remains a major challenge.

Inadequate Financial Resources and a Decentralized Fiscal System Impede Social Service Provision

Weak policy implementation is also related to current financing levels and mechanisms. For poor populations, the financial resources allocated for child welfare and child protection assistance are currently insufficient to meet their basic living standards. Also, as discussed above, China's highly decentralized fiscal system obliges local governments to supplement central-level fiscal transfers and to pay for basic social services and assistance at local levels, such as cash transfers for *dibao* or medical financial assistance payments. The lack of financial resources at lower administrative levels, especially poor counties and villages, is a major barrier to the universal provision of basic social services at community level. Since the level of social assistance is highly dependent on the local government's fiscal capacity, there are significant variations and inequalities across the country in terms of access to social services. Poor households in impoverished areas are therefore less likely to receive basic assistance or social services to meet minimum living standards (Dollar, 2007).

Sustainability of Protection Systems in an Economic Downturn

The Chinese government has greatly increased its spending on social services, including those for children, in recent years. This has occurred in an environment in which the economy and the government's overall fiscal resources have been expanding rapidly, meaning that these expenditures have been made without having to cut back on other government programs. At present, there are increasing concerns about the sustainability of China's rapid growth due to both international uncertainty and domestic risks. It is not clear that the current social protection programs will function as an effective social safety net if the economy enters a downturn and government revenues are affected. Social protection and social services are most urgently needed by poor households during a period of economic decline, and yet this has to be set against the great pressure placed on government to direct funds and support productive economic sectors. Thus, the sustainability of social services and social protection in a downturn would require a degree of advanced institutionalization and rules-driven budget allocations, both of which need further development in China.

Fragmented Systems and Vertical Institutional Structures Undermine Necessary Coordination

Given the legacy of the single-issue approach to social welfare and child protection programs in China, the social welfare, child protection, and justice systems and corresponding programs remain fragmented, with a continued reactive focus on issues or categories of children. Current child protection interventions also focus more on response than on prevention. Moving beyond individual schemes and vertical programs and increasing the focus of interventions on the prevention and the reduction of risks for children would greatly support better outcomes for children, and a more integrated, cost-effective child welfare and protection system and interventions.

In addition, there is a continued absence of integrated, coordinated linkages between sectors, particularly between the health, education, and child protection sectors, at various levels, including national, provincial, and community levels. In many countries, for example, health workers and teachers at the community level are required to screen for disability, abuse, neglect, or families at risk and report any findings to community social workers. Social workers then go on to investigate and provide appropriate services, family support, and referrals for more specialized services, as required. Social welfare support to families would be greatly enhanced by first establishing a national coordination body with an authoritative mandate to facilitate multisectoral cooperation and then developing mechanisms to support policy implementation at various levels, such as public financing allocations and governance systems regulating local intersectoral implementation.

Tendency to Expand Institutions for Children without Parental Care

The Chinese government's issues-based approach to child protection is also manifested in associated institutions for children without caregivers. SWIs, CWIs, and SCPCs provide long-term support and residential care for orphaned children, including children affected by HIV/AIDS, abandoned children (including many children with disabilities), street children, and others without parental care. Based on international experience, placing children into residential institutions is considered to be a measure of last resort. The ideal forms of alternative care are kinship care, foster care, and community-based family-like care, which have been shown globally to be cost effective where effectively resourced, and to result in better outcomes in terms of the social, emotional, and healthy development of the child.

While CWIs recognize that kinship and foster care are better options than institutional care, there is a tendency in China to build and expand CWIs.

While the new 2011-2020 National Plan of Action for Children's Development positively calls for a minimum of one qualified child welfare professional in each community and a shelter for street children in each county and city, it also calls for the establishment of one CWI in each of these locales. It will be important for the government to discuss and determine the appropriate roles and responsibilities of these welfare institutions and SCPCs prior to expansion; this process should give some consideration to global lessons showing that institutional care is best used as a measure of last resort and for the shortest time possible. It will also be important to orient and incentivize institutions to support social work services that encourage family support, monitoring and case management; provide referral services; and facilitate alternative community-based care over institutionalization.

In parallel, it will be important to work with existing CWIs, SWIs, and SCPCs in order to diversify their services, moving away from residential care and toward building systems for foster care and community-based solutions and placing children in alternative care in the best interests of each child. It will also be essential to tailor social welfare policies and lower level implementation guidelines in the same vein in order to support community-based alternative care. For example, the new orphan subsidy supports kinship and foster care. However, the subsidy for institutions (1,000 RMB) is greater than that for kinship and foster care (600 RMB), and this may have the unintended effect of creating incentives to institutionalize orphaned children rather than to seek alternative care options for them. The implementing regulations, for example, would benefit from a delineation of the role of CWIs and clearer guidelines on how the orphan subsidy to institutions can be used to facilitate alternative community-based care.

Nascent Child Welfare and Child Protection System in China

In addition, the child welfare system in China is still in its early stages of development. Current trends—rapid economic growth, large-scale migration, urbanization, changing family structures—will increase children's vulnerability to new risks, and the existing social welfare and protection system will not be able to prevent and respond to these risks completely. Social security and child protection systems will need to be significantly bolstered. In particular, the low availability and unequal access to community-based public social services, especially family support and child protection for the most vulnerable, will need to be addressed.

Social Work System in Early Stages of Development

The social work field is still a nascent profession in China, and the number of qualified social workers is currently very low. In 2009, only 8,418 people were certified as professional social workers and about 27,000 people were certified as social worker assistants. Moreover, the majority of these professionals have not yet had the opportunity to gain social work experience. With a population of over 1.3 billion, China needs an estimated 10 million social workers. According the government's national human resources development plan, China aims to have 2 million social workers by 2015 (State Council, 2010). However, it will be many years before a professional corps of qualified social workers is established and operational to meet welfare needs in China.

Underdeveloped Nonprofit Sector for Providing Community-based Social Services

Across the world, social welfare provision often encompasses a mix of interventions provided by the public, private, and nonprofit sectors. Each country needs to determine what mix is best for it at different stages of its development. As mentioned above, in a positive move, the Chinese government plans to expand the number of social work positions in the public sector and is experimenting with government procurement of nonprofit social work services. However, China's nonprofit sector could be further developed given the enormous potential of this sector to help meet the significant need for community-level social welfare services and to alleviate social problems at their root. Exploring further avenues for expanding nonprofit-sector social welfare services will be important for the development of more effective overall social service provision in the country, particularly in rural areas where the needs are greatest. At the same time, it will be important to ensure adequate registration, regulation and inspection, supported by national standards, training and guidance materials.

Specifically, it will be essential to provide an enabling environment for the development of the nonprofit sector. This would include simplifying the registration process and reducing the registration requirements for nonprofit organizations. At the same time, for both the nonprofit sectors and the public and private sectors, it will be important to establish adequate regulatory frameworks to support accountability and transparency in the management and use of donated funds and to develop monitoring and evaluation frameworks for social work service standards and implementation. These measures will be critical to supporting the effective management of social services and positive social welfare outcomes for children.

Unequal Access to Public Social Services for Children

Despite national efforts to increase social protection and service access, ensuring good coverage and equitable access to services for all remains a challenge; for the 211 million migrants in China, in particular, significant barriers exist. Access to social welfare provision is still hampered by policy and structural constraints intrinsic to the provision of social benefits under the existing *hukou* system. For example, RCMS benefits, among many others, are still not transferrable to urban areas, and so many poor migrants are still unable to afford health care and have to forego some primary health care services due to cost. Despite guarantees of 9 years of free compulsory education, a large percentage of migrant children do not attend public school. Vulnerable children left in rural areas by migrating parents are exposed to increased risks of trafficking, abuse, and exploitation. As previously mentioned, a UNICEF-supported CDPF survey showed that 61% of children with disabilities had not received the benefits aimed for them, including medical assistance, rehabilitation, educational subsidies or fee reductions, and vocational training (China Disabled Persons' Federation,

2006). There is a great need to support universal coverage of essential services in policy as well as in practice.

Large Number of Unregistered Children without Access to Social Services

Beyond those who do have access to public social services, it is likely that a significant number of children in China are unregistered and therefore do not have access to public services and protection. In order to access basic rights to health, education, social welfare, assistance, and protection under the law in China, a child must have a birth registration and a *hukou* (household registration). There are no current birth registration statistics in China. The most recent statistics available are from 1991 to 1999, and these show that during this period, only 60 to 80 per cent of children were registered within a year of their birth (Plan, 2011). There are over 340 million children in China. If between 20 to 40 per cent of births are unregistered, this would imply that an extremely large number of children are unable to access basic social services and social protection. Other research has indicated that the birth registration rate is low, particularly in poor and remote areas, for girls, migrant children, adopted children, and children born outside of locally sanctioned family planning limits, with some overlap among these categories (Li, 2009). Unregistered children are therefore especially vulnerable.

V. UNICEF SUPPORT TO STRENGTHEN CHINA'S CHILD WELFARE AND CHILD PROTECTION SYSTEM

Child-friendly poverty reduction programs, labor and employment policies, and an essential package of health and education services are critical to preventing income poverty, meeting the essential needs of families and children, and reducing social protection risks. Over the past 30 years in China, UNICEF's Health, Nutrition, Education, Water and Environmental Sanitation, HIV/AIDS and Social Policy Programmes have been providing significant assistance to the Chinese government in these areas, promoting the healthy survival and development of children and helping the government to meet the essential needs of all children with equity. Toward this end, UNICEF assistance has helped to support child welfare policies and services that address the social inequalities, disadvantages, risks, and vulnerabilities of children and families in the general population. These interventions constitute primary prevention.

Equally critical are child welfare and child protection policies and services that reduce the risk of children experiencing violence, abuse, exploitation, and neglect. Children whose families are poor, who experience social exclusion due to discrimination or stigma, or who do not have parental care are more vulnerable to significant harm than their wealthier and more socially integrated peers. Vulnerable children include children living in poverty, children without caregivers, children with disabilities, children affected by HIV/AIDS, children whose parents are serving prison terms, children living on the streets, children in conflict with the law, child trafficking victims, children of migrant workers, children left behind in rural areas by migrating parents, and children with any combination of these or other difficult circumstances. Policies, services, and interventions targeted at reducing the risks associated with these vulnerable groups, families, and children are central to child protection work. UNICEF's Child Protection Programme has provided international experience and technical assistance to support these initiatives in China. These interventions focus on secondary and tertiary prevention (UNICEF-China, 2010).

The key UNICEF policy objectives for child welfare policy are therefore to 1) offset poverty, deprivation, vulnerability, social exclusion, and other risk factors that can lead to lifelong disadvantage; 2) promote and protect children's rights and healthy development; and 3) prevent and respond to abuse, neglect, exploitation, and violence (i.e., child protection) (UNICEF-China, 2010).

To help strengthen the child protection system, the key UNICEF goals over the next 5 years are first to strengthen upstream policy, legislative, and institutional frameworks for child protection system development, implementation, and monitoring; and second, to improve the availability and delivery of family support and community-based child protection services (UNICEF-China, 2010). Public awareness raising campaigns at national and local levels to promote positive social attitudes and behavior change will also be a significant feature of child protection programming.

To support the development of the child welfare and protection system in China, three main levels of support will be provided to the government: 1) strengthening child welfare and child protection system policies, laws, and frameworks at the upstream and national level; 2) implementing national policies and laws at the intermediate and provincial level; and 3) piloting integrated child welfare and child protection models at the community level (feeding into upstream policies and intermediate implementation). This includes supporting the development of social work capacity.

A. Policies and Laws at the Upstream National Level

Upstream Child Welfare System Support

At the upstream level, it will be important to support China in improving its national strategies, laws, legal frameworks, policies, and plans and moving toward the provision of a comprehensive child welfare system. This will not only include providing policy analysis and technical input to assist the development of child welfare policies, laws, and frameworks (e.g., the Child Welfare Act), but also providing support for the development of systems to ensure effective implementation, such as a financing strategy to fund public functions and services, a human resources strategy (particularly for the social work system), multisectoral coordination mechanisms and networks, a service delivery system, a monitoring and evaluation mechanism, a cross-sectoral information system, a governance and accountability framework, and systems for implementing national standards and strategies.

National-level work also entails defining norms, standards, and costs for key aspects within the system, such as identifying the scope of public functions, defining a minimum package of services, costing minimum services across sectors, developing national child welfare standards, and supporting national-level advocacy and public awareness campaigns.

Foremost among China's child welfare policy frameworks are the 2011-2015 National Plan of Action for Child Welfare and the Child Welfare Act. Together, these are anticipated to outline the institutional, organizational, human resource, and financial aspects of the child welfare system, along with the scope of the expanded child welfare services.[8] The National Plan of Action for Child Welfare is expected to set out a broad vision for developing a child welfare system in China with a focus on strengthening family support and community-based services and diversifying and improving the services provided by CWIs (including daycare, respite care, outreach services, and the monitoring of children in kinship and foster care). The Child Welfare Act will (a) outline a broad legal framework for universal child welfare programs and assistance that goes beyond the current narrow focus on categories of vulnerable children and (b) aim to define the scope of diversified child welfare services (Institute of Social Development and Public Policy, 2008). It will be crucial to develop these frameworks with good technical support; UNICEF will support the Chinese government in this regard.

Over the past several years, UNICEF has supported various technical reviews and policy analyses that have contributed to the development of child welfare policy and legislative frameworks, strategies, national plans of actions, and implementation strategies. This assistance has included providing a comparative analysis of international and Chinese child welfare laws and policies, along with other technical social and economic policy analyses, and an analysis of child protection policies.

In the future, UNICEF will support additional policy analysis and technical assistance for the above frameworks. Importantly, UNICEF's experiences and evidence from empirical pilot work at various levels will also be analyzed and documented to inform upstream policymaking; for example, pilot experiences and feasibility analyses of implementing child welfare services at the community level in poor counties will be provided to inform policy development.

A multisectoral National Experts Group on Child Welfare System Policy and Legislative Development was established in 2010 to improve cross-sectoral coordination, initially for child welfare policy development. This group provides technical policy advice to the MCA on child welfare system development, and it will provide advice during the development of the new Five-year Plan of Action on Child Welfare (2011-2015) and the Child Welfare Act. It will also provide advisory inputs on the development of a minimum package of services and service standards. UNICEF will provide support by introducing international standards, norms, and experiences, and the MCA child welfare and protection pilots will support policy development with empirical evidence and data.

In support of a child welfare financing strategy, UNICEF is supporting the Ministry of Finance to undertake several studies to evaluate effective ways for financing the child welfare system. Research topics include improving financing for the rural and urban *dibao* systems, a policy study on financing early childhood development and equitable compulsory education for all, and research on government financing to support equalized public health services. UNICEF is also supporting the MCA in its efforts to define a minimum package of child welfare services and the scope of services and to undertake a costing for community-based services in different socioeconomic settings. These will feed into the larger child welfare financing strategy.

---

[8] This will include the legislative, regulatory, and policy frameworks; the effective enforcement of laws and regulations to protect children; adequately staffed and funded child protection services; intersectoral coordination and referral mechanisms to ensure that child welfare is supported by all public services; and public awareness and family education services to support positive social behaviors and good parenting practices.

According to a 2010 State Council Personnel Development Plan, China aims to have 2 million qualified social workers by 2015 (State Council, 2010) and to place one qualified social worker in every community at the rural township and urban subdistrict level. Given China's incipient social work system, the MCA will develop a new Five-year Plan for the Development of Social Work for Children which will help to develop a human resources strategy for a comprehensive child welfare system. In the coming years, UNICEF will provide technical assistance to help the MCA to develop (a) social worker positions in the public and nonprofit sectors, (b) national social work guidelines and standards for the professional qualification of social workers, (c) methodologies for evaluating social work services for children, (d) a national policy on government purchase of nonprofit social work services, and (e) related guidelines for nonprofit social welfare organizations.

To facilitate improved national monitoring and evaluation systems, the MCA and UNICEF are working together to develop a child vulnerability monitoring mechanism to provide timely identification, prevention, and response support to at-risk children. The MCA is also developing a case management database on social assistance and a system for carrying out periodic analyses of urban and rural medical financial assistance.

In addition, monitoring and evaluating the effectiveness of implementation mechanisms for social assistance policies will be another key area of support. A study on the implementation mechanism for disbursing the new cash transfer to orphans and for assessing the impact of the subsidy on recipients was initiated. The MCA is also working with UNICEF to examine the feasibility of incorporating a child poverty component into the current *dibao* scheme and to undertake policy research on (a) the intergenerational transmission of poverty in urban *dibao* families, (b) improved modalities to link child social assistance recipients with social work services, and (c) stronger linkages between the basic medical insurance and medical financial assistance to increase health coverage and social protection.

In support of increasing public awareness on child welfare issues, government partners will conduct various national information campaigns, ranging from high-profile advocacy events to sustained education and communication initiatives on child welfare related issues.

Upstream Child Protection System Support

UNICEF will be providing support to the various national government partners on the aspects of children protection policy described below.

To support cross-sectoral collaboration in the child protection system in China, several reference documents were developed for the government, including an international review outlining of the social and economic costs of child maltreatment and the comparative benefits of a national child protection system and a study on the legal and policy framework of China's child protection system. In the future, the government will convene meetings for key child protection system actors at national and local level to discuss and develop a vision for a comprehensive national child protection system across sectors. To lay the groundwork for these discussions, the NWCCW is undertaking a mapping and an analysis of child protection laws, policies, and services in China and the key responsibilities among various governmental departments. This mapping will help to identify gaps and areas where intersectoral linkages could be strengthened and to develop a continuum of policies and services for vulnerable children. A needs and cost analysis on the provision of child protection services will also be conducted by China's National Development and Reform Commission to guide strategic planning for developing the child welfare and protection system.

In addition, UNICEF will support the government to initiate child protection bodies to improve (a) the development, implementation, and enforcement of child protection policies and laws and (b) multisectoral coordination for child protection services delivery. Supporting government reforms in the justice system to improve the protection of child victims, witnesses, and offenders; to promote restorative justice models; and to strengthen data collection and knowledge management for evidence-based systems development are also key programming areas.

Violence against children. To improve the laws protecting children from violence and abuse, UNICEF is sharing international standards and best practices, supporting data collection, and facilitating multisectoral discussion on violence against children. UNICEF's work includes providing support to the National People's Congress and the All-China Women's Federation to study and promote the development of a new Law on Family Violence. Under this proposed legislation, key areas of advocacy will include a multisectoral approach to preventing and responding to violence (including mandatory reporting by professionals such as health workers, teachers, and social workers) and defining family violence to include children witnessing domestic violence. The government is also developing working procedures with clearly defined responsibilities and cooperation mechanisms across sectors to assist child victims of various forms of violence.

Trafficking. With respect to antitrafficking efforts, the government is developing its next National Plan of Action on Combating Trafficking in Women and Children (2013-2017), the aim of which is to improve coordination across government sectors. The government will also undertake a comparative legal analysis and review to identify gaps between national legislation and the Palermo Protocol. UNICEF will provide technical assistance during the development of the NPA and the legal analysis. China signed MOUs with Myanmar in 2009 and with Vietnam in 2010 in order to prevent and combat cross-border trafficking. In the coming years, UNICEF will further support the development of additional antitrafficking MOUs between China and neighboring countries.

China plans to conduct a technical legislative review of the Criminal Code to review the definition of child trafficking, including the age of the child and exemptions from criminal liability for victims of trafficking. In addition, the government will develop child-friendly national service guidelines to assist victims of trafficking and improve investigation procedures for child trafficking victims and working procedures for assisting child victims of violence. Good practices from the ACWF-UNICEF pilot initiative on the prevention of trafficking will feed into policy development for further prevention work.

Juvenile Justice. After the government revised the Law on the Protection of Minors and the Criminal Law, China adopted policies and regulations to protect children and youths in conflict with the law, established specialized departments and juvenile courts to handle juvenile cases, and began piloting noncustodial practices and child-friendly investigation and court procedures. To support a more child-centered juvenile justice system, UNICEF will provide assistance in three key areas over the next several years: (1) research to contribute to evidence-based policy and legislative development, including research on child-friendly trial procedures to protect child victims, witnesses, and offenders; (2) promotion of restorative justice models and community-based rehabilitation for children in conflict with the law to divert child offenders from the formal judicial system; and (3) introduction of international standards and best practices into juvenile justice, including the dissemination of internationally developed juvenile justice indicators to guide lawyers, judges, and juvenile justice workers.

Data and research. Over the next year, in order to improve the availability of data and analysis on key child protection areas, UNICEF is supporting the development of a national data monitoring system for children with disabilities; research on violence against children; a study on the psychosocial support needs of vulnerable children; and research to identify the major barriers to implementing child protection laws and policies. Data analysis will help support the government in its efforts to improve policies and program interventions, particularly those designed to prevent violence against children and the abuse and exploitation of children.

B. Implementation of Policies and Laws at the Intermediate or Provincial Level

Given China's large population and multilayered, financially decentralized structure, it is essential to provide support to ensure effective policy implementation and service delivery at lower levels. Thus, at the intermediate level, UNICEF assistance focuses on supporting provincial-level and midlevel implementation of national strategies, policies, laws, standards, rules, and regulations on child welfare and child protection and on building the capacity at provincial level to improve family and community care services for poor and vulnerable children. This includes supporting the development of (a) provincial-level financing strategies covering both provincial budget allocations and payment mechanisms, (b) a provincial human resources strategy for social workers, (c) monitoring and accountability systems, (d) integrated information systems, (e) planning and management tools, and (f) public awareness campaigns on child welfare.

With the launch of China's new 2011-2011 National Plan of Action for Children's Development, UNICEF will support the government to implement the NPA at lower administrative levels in the coming years, particularly the child welfare and child protection components, along with various aspects of the policies and laws discussed in the section above. More immediately, UNICEF will support the MCA's efforts to design and pilot the implementation of a medical financial assistance policy to support poor segments of the population suffering from severe diseases. UNICEF will also support the government to conduct training workshops on the design and implementation of child-sensitive social assistance programs. To increase awareness at the intermediate level, provincial public awareness campaigns supporting a child-friendly child welfare and protection system will be carried out.

C. Piloting Child Welfare and Child Protection Models at the Community Level

Over the next 5 years, UNICEF will be assisting the government to pilot community-based child welfare and child protection service models targeting the poorest and the most vulnerable children. At the community level, key aspects of an effective service model include a package of public services, a well-developed network of family support and community-based child protection services to protect children from significant harm, and strong social work services to identify and protect the most vulnerable children and families. In general, a well-developed child-friendly social protection system should provide a range of social and child welfare services, including family and social support services, child protection services, and alternative care.

The main goal of developing these models is to demonstrate cost-effective, and sustainable child welfare and child protection models for potential government replication. The lessons and insights gained from empirical pilot experiences will be documented and will contribute to the development of both upstream policy frameworks and downstream service guidelines, standards, and inspection mechanisms. Together, they will help to improve national child welfare policies and systems development and support effective service delivery in communities.

One model being piloted includes the development of child-sensitive approaches to social protection. UNICEF is currently collaborating with the MCA to pilot categorized social assistance schemes for children under the *dibao* system in urban areas and cash transfer models linking vulnerable child recipients to community-based social services such as health and education services. This approach involves UNICEF support to help the MCA study the implementation and monitoring mechanisms of the new orphan subsidy policy.

Another model being piloted is the Child Welfare Demonstration Pilots currently being carried out in counties with large numbers of children affected by AIDS (as described in Part III). The empirical evidence gained from developing and implementing both a universal package of child welfare services for all children at risk and a package of child protection services aimed at protecting children from discrimination, stigma, and significant harm will make an important contribution to policy development.

In a different model being piloted, UNICEF is working closely with the MCA to pilot and develop an integrated model for community-based child welfare services in vulnerable rural communities. In light of the vulnerability of children left behind in rural areas by migrating parents, this model is being piloted in areas with large numbers of such children, although services are available to all vulnerable children.

UNICEF is also supporting the government to develop a model for comprehensive community-based child protection services. This model will focus on establishing effective family support and community-based mechanisms and services to prevent children being subjected to violence, abuse, neglect and exploitation, including trafficking, sexual exploitation, and labor exploitation, and to monitor, identify, report, refer, and assist those children who are at risk of or have suffered these forms of harm. Associated social work services include monitoring poor and vulnerable children in the community, case management, home visits, counseling, referrals, and the facilitation of alternative care options as needed. The CPUs being piloted in four counties and the 30 CFS models in Sichuan (discussed in Part III) demonstrate aspects of this model.

Given the current institutional childcare structures in China, the support provided to the MCA to diversify the range of services offered in CWIs and SCPCs is important. Therefore, the MCA is beginning to diversify and expand the services offered by SCPCs in urban areas, as illustrated earlier by the Zhengzhou Model, and to pilot temporary shelter services for vulnerable children.

The MCA is also beginning to expand community-based alternative care options. Thus, UNICEF is supporting the MCA to pilot alternative care practices for vulnerable children, including foster care and community-based family-like care (e.g., daycare centers, family-based long-term care) for children without parental care and children with disabilities. At the same time, UNICEF will support programs to prevent family separation. The intention of the alternative care model is to meet the needs of all vulnerable children requiring such care, including children affected by HIV/AIDS, children with disabilities, orphaned and abandoned children, children living on the streets, and children without parental care. A key goal of the alternative care pilot schemes is to demonstrate that community-based care is not only better for the survival and the lifelong development of these children, as shown by international experience, but also that alternative care is cost effective and more sustainable in comparison to institutional care.

To support the effective implementation of all of these models, technical assistance is being provided to build the capacity of child protection professionals and community workers. UNICEF is also supporting the development of service guidelines and modules for daycare centers, positive discipline, and psychosocial support training for community workers and school teachers.

These models will also be strengthened by more clearly defined institutional frameworks, including goals, roles, and responsibilities; institutional arrangements; provisions for supporting sustainability; and government financing.

To promote positive social attitudes and behaviors that support the realization of children's rights and contribute to their healthy development, UNICEF will work with government partners to support public awareness, social mobilization, and advocacy campaigns.

These campaigns will help to increase awareness and knowledge of practices that are harmful and practices that are beneficial to children. They will highlight the issues faced by particularly vulnerable children (such as street children, orphans, children with disabilities, trafficked children), violence against children, and the value of family support and community-based services and care.

To monitor the impact of these campaigns and changes in terms of awareness and knowledge of, and social attitudes and behaviors toward, children, UNICEF will undertake surveys on knowledge, practices, and attitudes in the coming years.

CONCLUSION

Having taken the initial steps to reforming its social welfare system policies and services, China is making progress toward developing a more integrated child welfare and child protection system.

The Chinese government is moving toward more universalist approaches to social welfare for families and children, for example, by expanding social assistance programs such as *dibao* and medical financial assistance support, widening health insurance coverage and medical financial assistance, and supporting free compulsory education. While there is a continued tendency to focus on categories of children, the government is also encouraging more multisectoral approaches to specific child protection issues (e.g., by developing intersectoral NPAs to combat trafficking and to assist street children). To meet the emerging child welfare and protection challenges and to better protect children from significant harm from violence, abuse, exploitation, and neglect, the government will need to further strengthen and deepen the integration of the child welfare and protection system.

Specifically, the government will need to overcome various factors constraining the development of an effective child welfare and protection system. Supporting universal benefits for basic child welfare provisions will be instrumental in reducing unequal access to public social services for children and their families.

Increased central-level financial inputs for child welfare and child protection into areas with lower fiscal capacity, combined with more effective and efficient financing mechanisms for the use of funds, are greatly needed. In particular, improving enforcement measures and strengthening local-level accountability frameworks for public officials to provide public social services would significantly enhance actual access to services for vulnerable children and greatly improve policy implementation.

Vertical government structures and institutional arrangements will need to be further integrated. A national coordination body and improved intersectoral coordination mechanisms at different levels that help to promote a continuum of policies and services addressing the needs of vulnerable children would greatly facilitate meaningful integration.

Social workers have a critical role to play. To meet the current large gap in social work provision, the government will need to accelerate the development of the social work system and increase the number of trained social workers available at the national, provincial and community level. Importantly, facilitating the expansion of the nonprofit sector and other private social work agencies to contribute to the provision of social work services would help to relieve the great demand and need for social work services.

While the child welfare and child protection system in China is still developing, the government has already demonstrated its commitment to promoting child rights and has begun to address some of the barriers mentioned above. In the coming years, UNICEF will continue to support the government to develop a more comprehensive child welfare and protection system by providing policy and legislative inputs for child welfare and child protection systems development, strengthening capacity at national, provincial, and local levels, piloting approaches for evidence-based policy development and legislative reform, and undertaking communication campaigns for positive social change for children. UNICEF will continue to play a supporting role by introducing international best practices, standards, and norms for the government to consider and adapt as appropriate to the Chinese context.

ACKNOWLEDGMENTS

I am grateful to David Hipgrave, William Bikales, Etienne Poirot, Chen Xuemei, and Diane Swales for their insightful reviews. I would also like to express my appreciation to the Social Policy, Child Protection, and HIV/AIDS Teams of UNICEF-China for developing the initial UNICEF conceptual program frameworks to support child welfare and child protection systems in China, particularly Hana Brixi, Chen Xuemei, Kirsten Di Martino, Huang Jinxia, Mu Yan, Etienne Poirot, Shi Weilin, Wang Daming, Xu Wenqing, Yang Haiyu, and Zhang Lei.

APPENDIX

Acronyms

ACWF	All-China Women's Federation
BMI	Basic Medical Insurance
CDPF	China Disabled Persons' Federation
CFS	Child friendly space
CPU	Child protection unit
CRC	Convention on the Rights of the Child
CWI	Child welfare institution
EAPRO	East Asia and the Pacific Regional Office (UNICEF)
ECD	Early childhood development
EPI	Expanded Programme on Immunization
GDP	Gross domestic product
MCA	Ministry of Civil Affairs
MFA	Medical Financial Assistance
MOE	Ministry of Education
MOH	Ministry of Health
MOU	Memorandums of understanding
NBS	National Bureau of Statistics
NCMS	New Cooperative Medical Scheme
NPFPC	National Population and Family Planning Commission
NPA	National Plan of Action
NWCCW	National Working Committee on Women and Children
RCMS	Rural Cooperative Medical Scheme
RMB	Ren min bi (official currency of China)
SWI	Social welfare institution
SCPC	Street children protection center
UNICEF	United Nations Children's Fund
UNFPA	United Nations Population Fund
URBMI	Urban Resident Basic Medical Insurance
WHO	World Health Organization

REFERENCES

Brixi, H. (2009). *China: Urban services and governance.* China: UNICEF.

Brixi, H., Mu, Y., Targa, B., and Hipgrave, D. (2011). *Equity and public governance in health system reform: Challenges and opportunities for China.* (Forthcoming publication.)

Chen, J., Dai, D., Pu, M., Hou, W., and Feng, Q. (2010). *The trend of the Gini coefficient in China.* BWPI Working Paper 109, Brooks World Poverty Institute, University of Manchester. Retrieved from http://www.bwpi.manchester.ac.uk/resources/Working-Papers/bwpi-wp-10910.pdf

Chen, S., and Ravallion, M. (2008). *China is poorer than we thought, but no less successful in the fight against poverty,* World Bank Policy Research Working Paper 4621. Washington DC: World Bank.

China Development Research Foundation. (2007). *China development report 2007: Eliminating poverty in development.* Beijing.

China Disabled Persons' Federation. (2006). *Second national sample survey of disability.* Beijing.

China Health Economics Institute. (2006). *China national health account report.* China.

Chinese Center for Disease Control and Prevention. (2005). *China food and nutrition surveillance report.* China.

Di Martino, K., Weilin, S., and Xuemei, C. (2010). *Developing a comprehensive child welfare system in China.* UNICEF background paper for the 2010 High-Level Meeting on International Cooperation for Child Rights.

Dollar, D. (2007). *Poverty, inequality and social disparities during China's economic reform.* China: World Bank.

Duan, C., and Zhou, F. (2005). Research on China's left-behind children. *Population Research, 29:29-36.*

The Economist. (2010, March 4). Gendercide: The worldwide war on baby girls: Technology, declining fertility and ancient prejudice are combining to unbalance societies. Retrieved from http://www.economist.com/node/15636231.

Edlund, L., Li, H., Yi, J., and Zhang, J. (2007). *Sex ratios and crime: Evidence from China's one-child policy.* IZA Discussion Paper Series 3214, Institute for the Study of Labor. Berlin.

Evaluation Task Force for NCMS. (2006). *Evaluation report on NCMS piloting counties.* Beijing: People's Health Publishing House.

Institute of Social Development and Public Policies, Beijing Normal University. (2008). *Study on the child welfare system in China.* Beijing: Child Welfare Centre.

Li, S., Zhang, Y., and Feldman, M. (2009). Birth registration in China: Practices, problems and policies. *Population Research and Policy Review, 29,* 297-317.

Ministry of Civil Affairs. (2009 and 2010). *China civil affairs statistical yearbook 2009 and 2010.* Retrieved from http://www.mca.gov.cn/article/zwgk/mzyw/201106/ 20110600 161364.shtml

Ministry of Education, National Bureau of Statistics, Ministry of Finance. (2010). *The 2009 statistical notice on national education expenditure.* Beijing.

Ministry of Education of China. (2009). *Essential statistics of education in China.* China.

Ministry of Foreign Affairs of the People's Republic of China and the UN System in China. (2010). *China's progress towards the millennium development goals: 2010 report.* Retrieved from http://www.un.org.cn/cms/p/resources/30/1539/content.html

Ministry of Health. (2009). *China health statistical yearbook.* China.

Ministry of Health. (2010). *China health statistical yearbook.* Beijing: China Union Medical University Press.

National Bureau of Statistics. (2005). *2008 China population.* China.

National Bureau of Statistics. (2007). *One per cent population sample survey.* China (2005 data).

National Bureau of Statistics of China. (2008). *National sample survey on population.* China: China Statistics Press.

National Bureau of Statistics of China. (2010). *2010 China statistical yearbook.* China.

National Population and Family Planning Commission. (2010). *The 2010 report on the development of China's floating population.* China.

Office of Migrant Workers of the State Council and All China Women's Federation. (February 2008). *Research report on rural left-behind children in China.* China.

Peking University. (2005). *Retrospective survey on childhood violence experiences among young people in China.* Beijing.

Plan International. (2011). *Universal birth registration: Country case studies: China.* Retrieved from http://plan-international.org/birthregistration/resources/country-case-studies/china

Shang, X., and Xiaolin, W. (2011). *China's child welfare update, discovery report: Emerging issues and findings for child welfare and protection in China.* China: Social Sciences Academic Press.

Shang X., Xiaolin, W., and Jing, T. C. (2010). *Survival children, discovery report: Emerging issues and findings for child welfare and protection in China. Research on the reform of state child welfare institutions.* China: Social Science Academic Press.

State Council of the People's Republic of China. (2006). *Some opinions to address the issues of rural migrant workers.* China.

State Council of the People's Republic of China. (2010). *Outline of the national medium and long term program for personnel development (2010-2020).* Beijing: State Council of the People's Republic of China.

State Council of the People's Republic of China. (2011). *National plan of action for children's development, 2011-2020.*

Tsai, L. (2007). *Accountability without democracy: Solidarity groups and public good provision in rural China.* Cambridge and New York: Cambridge University Press.

UNFPA. (2010). *State of the world's population 2010, from conflict and crisis to renewal: Generations of change.* New York.

UNICEF. (2008). *Child protection strategy.* New York.

UNICEF. (2009). *2009 State of the world's children.*

UNICEF-China. (2008). *Mid-term review of UNICEF contribution towards health and nutrition improvement strategies in China, 2006-2008.* Beijing, China.

UNICEF-China. (2010). *China Country Programme Document (2011-2015).* Beijing.

UNICEF-China (2010). *Conceptual framework for the development of a child welfare system in China.* Beijing. (Internal UNICEF working document).

UNICEF East Asia and the Pacific Regional Office. (2009). *East Asia and the Pacific child protection programme strategy toolkit.* Bangkok: UNICEF EAPRO.

United Nations. (1989). Convention on the Rights of the Child. Retrieved 15 November 2011 from http://www2.ohchr.org/english/law/crc.htm#art19.

Waldmeir, P. (2011, July 27). China cracks down on child kidnappings. *Financial Times.* Retrieved from: http://www.ft.com/intl/cms/s/0/3909b53e-b857-11e0-8d23-00144 feabdc0.html#axzz1Z2SAasCT

World Bank (2006). *Health reform in rural China: Where next?* Washington, DC: World Bank.

World Bank. (2009). *From poor areas to poor people: China's evolving poverty reduction agenda: An assessment of poverty and inequality in China.* Washington, DC: World Bank.

World Health Organization. (2009). *Global health observatory data repository.* Geneva, Switzerland.

Xinhua News Agency. (2011, August 17). Millions of Chinese men without brides by 2020 due to gender imbalance: Experts warn. Retrieved from http://news.xinhuanet.com/english2010/china/2011-08/17/c_131056376.html.

In: Child Welfare
Editors: Alex Powell and Jenna Gray-Peterson
ISBN: 978-1-62257-826-9
© 2013 Nova Science Publishers, Inc.

Chapter 7

MINDFULNESS TRAINING: A PROMISING APPROACH FOR ADDRESSING THE NEEDS OF CHILD WELFARE SYSTEM CHILDREN AND FAMILIES

Cynthia V. Heywood, Philip A. Fisher and Yi-Yuan Tang
Oregon Social Learning Center, University of Oregon,
Eugene, Oregon, US

ABSTRACT

Foster children often demonstrate intensive clinical needs and evidence risk for long-term difficulties as a result of adversity and maltreatment. Addressing their diverse and intensive needs can be challenging for foster caregivers and complex for their providers. Although intervention research over the past decades has yielded a number of evidence-based treatment approaches for foster children and their caregivers, enhancement and individualization continues to be needed.

As the field advances, more attention is being paid to critical skills that increase competence and resilience as protective factors versus the more traditional focus on pathology. Particularly, self-regulation and attention are becoming increasingly salient foci for scientists and practitioners seeking to improve treatment effectiveness and favorable outcomes.

Mindfulness-oriented interventions pose a forum for uniquely targeting these outcomes and have the potential to (1) promote the development of self-regulation and attentional focus in foster children, (2) increase the effect of already robust therapies, (3) enhance risk prevention efforts for children whose lives are characterized by adversity, (4) address obstacles to effective and consistent implementation of therapeutic parenting strategies, and (5) increase overall well-being and quality of life for foster children and their caregivers. In this chapter, the following topics are discussed: (1) the presenting issues among foster children and their need for effective and individualized treatments, (2) the interplay of stress and neurobiology on the development critical skills, (3) current intervention trends, and (4) applications for mindfulness-oriented therapies in research and practice.

The presence of over one-half million children in out-of-home care in the United States represents a national public health concern given that the vast majority of these placements result from abuse or neglect (Kendall, Dale, and Plakitsis, 1995; Stein, 1997). Over the past 20 years, the foster care population has grown considerably. Increases over time in the size of the foster care population, which until recently was growing by an average of 10% annually, are attributable to numerous factors. These include changes in child abuse and neglect reporting requirements, higher foster care entrance versus exit rates, and the impact of poverty, homelessness, adolescent parenthood, family violence, mental illness, and substance abuse. The issues are further exacerbated by flat or decreasing budgets for social services (Barbell, 1997; Barbell and Freundlich, 2001). In a national survey, states reported that funding for family support services has not kept pace with need, resulting in foster children languishing in care (U.S. General Accounting Office, 2007). As of 2008, there were more 463,000 foster children nationwide. Fortunately, the size of the population appears to have stabilized at around one-half million children in the past five years, and the most recent estimates indicate a decreasing trend (U.S. Department of Health and Human Services, 2009).

In this chapter, we will explore four areas related to foster children. First, we review the disparities in well-being among foster children. Second, we explore the impact of adversity and stress on specific neurodevelopmental processes that may help to account for some of these disparities. Third, we discuss current trends in intervention practices with foster children and their caregivers, emphasizing evidence-based interventions designed specifically for this population. Lastly, we explore a new trend in emotional and behavioral health with great promise for the foster care populations: specifically, interventions designed to impact the domain of mindfulness. We suggest that, given the unique sequelae resulting from maltreatment and early adversity, mindfulness-oriented treatments for foster children and their caregivers pose a unique and promising approach for remediating critical deficits and addressing persistent obstacles to the implementation of more effective practices in the child welfare system.

PSYCHOSOCIAL, EMOTIONAL, AND ACADEMIC ADJUSTMENT IN FOSTER CHILDREN

Foster care is intended to interrupt the experience of chaos and stress that often typifies the lives of maltreated children and to provide a context in which the impact of this adversity can be ameliorated. Frequently, however, it takes multiple reports from community members before child welfare becomes involved and/or removes a child from their home. By this point, the child may have experienced a host of adversities which cumulatively have a profound and lasting impact on his/her development and well-being. The deleterious consequences of childhood maltreatment are well-documented in the literature and have been observed during childhood as well as across the lifespan. Consequently, providing a therapeutic foster care experience proves to be challenging and complex.

Despite the multitude of shared experiences that result in out-of-home placement, foster children demonstrate a wide array of outcomes with regard to psychosocial and emotional adjustment. It is important to note that there are many foster children who exhibit remarkable resilience in the face of considerable adversity. However, as a group, foster children are in much greater need of intervention for mental health problems than children in the general population (Chernofff, Combs-Orme, Risley-Curtis, and Heiser, 1994; McIntyre and Thomas, 1986; Pilowsky, 1995). Specifically, foster children have high rates of internalizing problems (e.g., anxiety disorders, depressive symptomotology, dissociative disorders, somatic complaints, eating disorders, and suicidal ideation), externalizing behavior disorders (e.g., aggression, delinquency, and antisocial behavior), attachment disorders, personality disorders, deficits in self-regulation, deficits in executive functioning, sexual reactivity, deficits in social competence, and difficulty forming healthy relationships with peers and adults (Ackerman et al., 1998; Bendixen, Muus, and Schei, 1994; Bolger and Patterson, 2003; Cicchetti and Toth, 1995; Hernandez, 1992; Kinard, 1999; Liem and Boudewyn, 1999; Mian, Marton, and LeBaron, 1996; Trickett and McBride-Chang, 1995; Weaver and Clum, 1993; Welch and Fairburn, 1996). Moreover, Dubowitz (1990) found that emotional, behavioral, and developmental difficulties among foster children were *three to six times greater* than those demonstrated among children within the general population. Trupin and colleagues found that 72% of child welfare children in their sample were not statistically unique from children participating in intensive mental health treatment programs (Trupin, Tarico, Low, Jennelka, and McClellan, 1993). Landsverk and Garland (1999) estimated that between one-half and two-thirds of all children entering the foster care system demonstrate emotional or behavioral problems significant enough to warrant mental health treatment. Clausen, Landsverk, Ganger, Chadwick, and Litrownik (1998) reported that 61% of their sample of foster children demonstrated clinically significant mental health problems as per the Child Behavior Checklist (Achenbach, 1991). Furthermore, the number of children coming into care demonstrates that these problems increased significantly over time during the 1980s and 1990s, highlighting the need for more comprehensive and effective service provision to address these concerns (U.S. General Accounting Office, 1998).

The risk for school problems is also greater among maltreated children. This is not surprising, given that the early caregiving environment provides the foundation for psychosocial adjustment integral to academic preparedness and success. Children with maltreatment histories have been shown to demonstrate significantly more deficits in academic engagement, social competence, and ego resiliency, resulting in overall academic maladjustment (Shonk and Cicchetti, 2001). Additionally, these children demonstrate higher rates of academic underachievement, grade retention, poor social competence, dropout, and utilization of special education services than their same-age peers (Rowe and Eckenrode, 1999; Trickett and McBride-Chang, 1995; Wodarski, Kurtz, Gaudin, and Howing, 1990). In a study of 840 children, Eckenrode, Laird, and Doris (1993) found that children who had been maltreated were significantly more likely to repeat a grade, have lower standardized test scores and grades, and receive higher rates of office discipline referrals and suspensions. Rogosch and Cicchetti (1994) examined teachers' perceptions of maltreated children and found that these students were seen as less socially competent than their peers and were perceived to exhibit greater behavioral disturbances in the classroom.

As noted above, problems with foster children's psychosocial, emotional and academic adjustment have been observed to extend well into adulthood. Skills decline over time, behavior patterns become entrenched, and ontogenic patterns become increasingly complex. For example, in a study of 900 victims of childhood abuse and neglect, Widom and Maxfield (2001) examined the effects on intellectual, behavioral, social, and psychological development into adulthood. Data revealed that, compared to a control group, the abused group scored significantly lower on measures of intellectual performance, completed fewer years of school, held more menial and semiskilled jobs, experienced higher rates of unemployment/underemployment, experienced higher rates of divorce and separation, engaged in higher rates of criminal behavior, and were more likely to demonstrate suicidality and personality disorders. The context often surrounding abuse, including parental criminality and substance abuse, coupled with childhood victimization increased the likelihood of later disorders.

Neurodevelopmental Deficits in Attention and Self-Regulation

Two underlying commonalities in the topography of negative sequelae described above are deficits in attention and self-regulation. These highly related constructs bear influence across a number of emotional and behavioral disorders. Exploring this relationship, however, first requires definitions of the constructs. Attention is a multifaceted capacity that entails three primary brain networks that carry out the functions of alerting (i.e., acquiring and maintaining an alert state), orienting (i.e., the reception of information from sensory input), and executive control (i.e., resolving conflict among thoughts, feelings, and responses; Posner and Dehaene, 1994; Rueda, Posner, and Rothbart, 2005). Self-regulation, as defined for these purposes, is comprised of two domains: emotional regulation (i.e., modulating affective states in response to fear and anger) and behavioral regulation (i.e., self-monitoring and inhibiting impulses). Physiological regulatory processes (e.g., sleep, arousal, and digestion) function as an important counterpart to self-regulation and will be discussed in greater detail below.

The emergence of self-regulation is a result of the executive function of attentional management and effortful control. When conflict between different neural networks occurs in response to a given stimulus, those neural networks compete for control, requiring the executive control system to govern the individual's response. For example, if an individual perceives an oncoming attack, the fight or flight response is activated. It is the executive control network that allows the individual to then determine how to respond: aggressively or in accordance with a different goal. The subsequent behavioral expression is a result of effortful control. Effortful control, defined as "the efficiency of executive attention, including the ability to inhibit a dominant response and/or to activate a subdominant response, to plan, and to detect errors," has been noted to play an integral role in the development of self-regulation (Rothbart and Bates, 2006), as it allows an individual to voluntarily shift attention, inhibit emotional responses, and modulate emotional and behavioral expression (Eisenberg et al., 2005). Many have argued that effortful control, as a component of emotion-related regulation, is an essential function of healthy emotional expression for minimizing lability and negativity (Eisenberg and Spinrad, 2006; Spinrad et al., 2006; Valiente, Lemery-Chalfant, Swanson, and Reiser, 2008).

Increasing attention has been paid to the role that self-regulation plays in a host of emotional and behavioral disorders, and researchers have found that deficits in this ability are associated with a multitude of psychopathologies (Barkley, 1997; Benton, 1991; Bradley, 2000; Cicchetti, Ackerman, and Izard, 1995; Davidson, 2000; Pennington, 1997). Self-regulation is an integral facet of externalizing behaviors, as hyperactivity, defiance, and aggression are all exemplified by a lack of inhibiting inappropriate behavior and modulating affective states. A number of researchers have demonstrated this link. For example, children found to have diminished effortful control have been noted as being more oppositional and less prepared for the classroom (Lewis, Dozier, Ackerman, and Sepulveda-Kozakowski, 2005). Rydell, Berlin, and Bohlin (2003) found that poor emotion regulation in early childhood predicted externalizing problem behaviors and decreased prosocial skills during middle childhood. The ability to regulate expressions of anger in young children has also been found to relate to chronic levels of covert antisocial behavior. Eisenberg and colleagues (2005) found that children demonstrating externalizing behavior problems were rated as lower in effortful control and higher in impulsivity. Researchers have also indicated that young children exhibiting aggression, poor affective regulation, and poor effortful control demonstrate strained relationships with teachers and peers and poor academic performance (Birch and Ladd, 1998; Valiente et al., 2008; Wentzel and Asher, 1995).

Attention has also proved to play a key role in internalizing behavior problems. Depression has been characterized by an inability to divert one's attention from a stressful stimulus or negative cognition (e.g., rumination), and this cognitive perseveration has been shown to predict later onset of anxiety and depression symptoms (Nolen-Hoeksema, 2000). Similarly, anxiety has been described an attentional bias to threat wherein the individual tends to allocate his/her attention to threat-relevant or emotionally negative cues (Bar-Haim, Lamy, Pergamin, Bakermans-Kranenburg, and van IJzendoorn, 2007; Beck, Emery, and Greenberg, 1985; Mogg and Bradley, 2005). Although much previous research in this area was correlational, the results from a recent study confirmed that attentional bias plays a causal role in the maintenance of Generalized Anxiety Disorder (Amir, Beard, Burns, and Bomyea, 2009). This attentional bias serves to increase the overall level of arousal in an individual resulting in stress-related dysfunction over time (Kiecolt-Glaser, McGuire, Robles, and Glaser, 2002; Salovey, Rothman, Detweiler, and Steward, 2000).

There have been surprisingly few studies on self-regulation or attention-related problems with specific regard to foster children. Children who are exposed to chaotic and unpredictable environments and stressors early in life, not unlike children with maltreatment histories, tend to exhibit anxiety that inhibits attentional focus because of heightened arousal and cognitive distortions (Vasey and Ollendick, 2000; Compas and Oppedisano, 2000). This is likely to be exacerbated under academic demands (Roeser and Eccles, 2000). Racusin, Maerlander, Sengupta, Straus, and Isquith (2003) found clinically significant deficits in inhibitory control, emotional modulation, and cognitive/behavioral flexibility among a considerable proportion of their sample of foster children with histories of trauma and disrupted attachment. Further, these deficits were strongly correlated with disordered attachments, behavior problems, psychiatric disorders, and diminished functioning. Slinning (2004) found that foster children exposed prenatally to substances but who were reared in low-risk care settings demonstrated significantly elevated levels of both impulsivity and attention problems, indicating a strong neurobiological basis of these behavior problems. Care settings, however, have also proved to play a role in the development of attention and self-regulation. In one study, compared to a community-based control group, children raised in substitute care (a combination of institutional and foster care) evidenced higher levels of hyperactivity and inattention continuously and beginning before 12 months of age (Roy, Rutter, and Pickles, 2000). Insufficient care and neglect appears to play a salient role in this regard. Pears and Fisher (2005) found that preschool-aged foster children with histories of neglect and emotional abuse scored significantly lower on executive functioning than foster children with other maltreatment subtypes (i.e., physical abuse or sexual abuse).

In spite of the relatively small number of studies discussed herein, given the critical involvement that self-regulation and attention play in a host of emotional and behavioral problems, it is likely that foster children evidence more deficits in functioning in these areas than their peers in the general population.

When functioning at more optimal levels, attentional focus and self-regulation can serve as protective factors that increase the likelihood of positive adaptation in the face of adversity. In their review of the development of emotion regulation, Morris, Silk, Steinberg, Myers, and Robinson (2007) argued that regulation is central to overall adjustment. The ability to modulate emotions and behavior in response to typical and novel stressors so as to respond in socially appropriate ways is integral not only to psychological adaptation but to the development of healthy relationships (Cicchetti et al., 1995; Denham et al., 2003). Additionally, the ability for a child to modulate emotional responses, behavior, and control impulses appropriately is vital to school adjustment; novel stressors and demands consistently emerge throughout childhood and adolescence (Birch and Ladd, 1998; Garon, Bryson, and Smith, 2008; Ladd, Birch, and Buhs, 1999; McClelland, Morrison, and Holmes, 2000). Dysregulation, therefore, places children at increased risk of exaggerated reactions to stressful events (Bruce, Davis, and Gunnar, 2002).

CURRENT INTERVENTION TRENDS

The Context for Care

The placement of a child in foster care is intended to be an intervention, and the removal of a child from their parents or primary caregivers, albeit traumatic, serves to suspend the adversity precipitating the involvement of child welfare. At the most basic level, foster caregivers shelter and protect the child for a period of time until a permanent placement plan is possible. At its best, foster care can potentiate healthy development in the child by placing them in a therapeutic context wherein foster caregivers can remediate skills on a multitude of domains. Additionally, it allows the child to experience himself/herself in the context of a normative family and to relearn a healthier caregiver–child dynamic, which can foster healthy attachment behaviors conducive to long-term care relationships. Concurrently during the child's placement out of home, biological parents or prior caregivers are subject to court mandates in the cases of abuse, neglect, and endangerment for the purpose of rehabilitation and skill remediation. Child welfare caseworkers monitor treatment, for both the child and the biological parents, and plan for permanency.

The time afforded to the foster child to accomplish these ends varies widely. In 2008, estimates of the length of stay in foster care indicated that 5% of foster children remained in care for less than 1 month, 37% remained in care for 1–11 months, 23% remained in care for 1–2 years, and 36% remained in care for more than 2 years (U.S. Department of Health and Human Services, 2009). More than half of all foster children were placed for less than 2 years; given the breadth and complexity of their treatment needs, this is a relatively brief time allotted for remediation before returning to what is often still an environment characterized by chaos and adversity. Of the near 285,000 children who exited foster care in 2008, 52% were reunited with parents or primary caregivers, 19% were adopted, 8% were placed with other relatives or family, 10% were emancipated, 7% were under the care of a legal guardian, and 3% had other outcomes (e.g., transfer to another agency and runaway; U.S. Department of Health and Human Services, 2009).

Instability (e.g., residential mobility, change of caregiver status, and a chaotic and unpredictable environment) is the hallmark of many of foster children's families of origin. This situation is not ameliorated, however, when a child enters foster care. Many foster children will move placements multiple times during out-of-home care. Researchers report that 22–56% of foster children have experienced three or more placements during their time in foster care (Newton, Litrownik, and Landsverk, 2000). Estimates for 2008 indicate the mean length of stay in foster care was 27.2 months (U.S. Department of Human Services, 2009). This is significant given that longer stays in the foster care system increase the likelihood of more placements, which decreases prospects for permanency (Barbell and Freundlich, 2001; Glisson, Bailey, and Post, 2000).

Foster children with behavior problems are more likely to experience disrupted placements and to be moved frequently, sometimes throughout the entirety of their childhood years. The disruptiveness of these volatile placement patterns contributes to internalizing and externalizing behavior problems in foster children (Newton et al., 2000). Similarly, the length of time in foster care and the number of placements have been linked to behavior problems and academic underachievement with a greater number of disruptions resulting in poorer outcomes (Benbenishty, and Oyserman, 1995; Zima et al., 2000). In general, family instability is significantly related to increased rates of negative emotionality, internalizing problem behaviors, and externalizing problem behaviors (Ackerman, Brown, and Izard, 2003; Ackerman, Brown, D'Eramo, and Izard, 2002; Ackerman, Kogos, Youngstrom, Schoff, and Izard, 1999). The risk for maladjustment due to family instability is moderated by child variables (i.e., temperamental adaptability and behavior and emotion regulation), meaning that children with lower levels of both demonstrate more adverse outcomes associated with family instability than their same-age peers (Ackerman et al., 1999). Psychosocial functioning is particularly important for young foster children because it significantly predicts the likelihood of reunification after out-of-home placements (Landsverk, Davis, Ganger, Newton, and Johnson, 1996). Similarly, volatile placement histories have also been shown to increase the risk of adoption disruption due to related problematic behavioral outcomes (Simmel, 2007). Further, instability compounds the negative consequences of abuse and neglect and significantly predicts outcomes across important areas of functioning such as school performance and self-regulation and the prevalence of internalizing and externalizing behavior problems (Ackerman et al., 2003; Ackerman et al., 2002; Newton et al., 2000).

In addition to behavioral maladjustment, number of placement transitions has been found to negatively correlate with executive function in preschoolers (Pears and Fisher, 2005), a critical component of school adjustment and functioning. Similarly, children who experienced multiple placement transitions during foster care were found to have lower inhibitory control and higher oppositional behavior once in their adoptive families (Lewis et al., 2007). This is likely explained by the negative impact of transition and stress on overall development (Gunnar, Fisher, and The Early Experience, Stress, and Prevention Network, 2006). In one study, academic skill delays were significantly predicted by number of out-of-home placements in that foster children with higher rates of placement disruptions were more likely to demonstrate at least one academic skill delay than foster children with more stable placement histories (Zima et al., 2000).

Treatment Approaches

The contextual complexities discussed above highlight the need for effective and targeted intervention support for foster children, their caregivers, and their families of origin. It is critical that these interventions not only address the emergent behavioral and emotional needs of the child but also serve to increase stability and successful permanency placements. Very few evidence-based interventions have been designed specifically for the foster care population. This is problematic because the unique constellation of needs among foster children presents distinctive challenges for treatment providers.

Two primary approaches have been employed for treatment in this population: (1) symptom-focused individual therapies principally targeted to the child, and (2) ecological and systems-focused interventions that address contextual factors that moderate child outcomes. Interventions with strong evidence bases that have been employed widely with this population and those specifically targeted to foster children are discussed below.

Symptom Reduction-Focused Interventions

Cognitive Behavioral Therapy (CBT). Underpinning the concept of CBT is the idea that thoughts (i.e., cognitions) influence emotion and behaviors. CBT is not a specific therapeutic technique per se but a way to classify a therapeutic approach. A number of reviews and studies have indicated the use of CBT as an effective intervention approach for treating depression, anxiety, conduct problems, impulsivity, suicidal ideation, and symptoms related to Post-Traumatic Stress Disorder (PTSD) in youth (Albano and Kendall, 2002; Asarnow, Jaycox, and Tompson, 2001; Baer and Neitzel, 1991; Lewinsohn, Clark, Rohde, Hops, and Seeley, 1996; Ollendick, 1998; Rotheram-Borus, Piacentini, Miller, Graae, and Castro-Blanco, 1994; Silverman, Kurtines, Ginsburg, Weems, Lumpkin, and Carmichael, 1999). CBT methods with youth encourage a constructive and problem-solving world view (Braswell and Kendall, 2003). This problem-solving orientation has also been referred to as a "coping template" supporting adaptive responses to stressors (Kendall and Panichelli-Mindel, 1995). Increasing self-awareness and teaching youth how to self-monitor their affective state is a common treatment element for youth demonstrating not only affective problems but also aggression (Nelson and Finch, 1996; Kendall, 1998; Kendall, 2000). However, given the highly verbal nature of this therapeutic approach, it is not well-suited to very young children. Currently, there is much debate in the field regarding use of CBT methods with clients who have intellectual disabilities (Taylor, Lindsay, and Willner, 2008).

Trauma-Focused CBT (TF-CBT). In certain cases where more severe trauma has been incurred as a result of abuse, TF-CBT may be indicated. In this approach, the basic principles of CBT as discussed above are augmented by an emphasis on gradual exposure that incrementally increases over the therapeutic relationship. Evidence for the use of TF-CBT with children is supported by a number of randomized control trials and effectiveness studies for survivors of sexual abuse, domestic violence, traumatic grief, disasters, terrorism, or multiple traumas (Celano and Rothbaum, 2002; Cohen, Deblinger, Mannarino, and Steer, 2004; Cohen and Mannarino, 2004; Cohen, Mannarino, Perel, and Staron, 2007; Feather and Ronan, 2006; Hoagwood et al., 2006; King et al., 2000). Parent involvement in TF-CBT can be particularly effective for children as reviewing traumatic events in the therapy setting can retrigger a host of negative affective experiences that must then be dealt with at home. Cohen and Mannarino (2008) discussed a model for joint parent–child treatment of TF-CBT for children ages 3–17 including the following components: psychoeducation and parenting skills, relaxation skills, affective regulation skills, cognitive coping skills, trauma narrative, and cognitive processing of the traumatic event(s), in vivo mastery of trauma reminders, conjoint child–parent sessions, and enhancing safety and future developmental trajectory.

Caregiver-Based Interventions

Behavioral Parent Training. U.S. federal policy indicates that all prospective foster parents receive sufficient training for meeting the needs of the child placed in their home (Foster Care Independence Act of 1999, H. R. 3443; English and Grasso, 1999). Specifications for practice, however, are determined at the state level. Generally, these include some form of parent training; however, the content, duration, and intensity of training are not standardized. Further complicating the matter, different training requirements exist for *treatment* foster caregivers who act as therapeutic agents and collaborate with other professionals to develop and implement treatment plans for the child (Chamberlain, 1994, 2002). In a review of current training practices and evidence for their effectiveness, Dorsey, Famer, Barth, Greene, Reid, and Landsverk (2008) noted that only 14 states require any additional preservice or annual inservice training hours for treatment foster caregivers. The guidelines set forth by the Foster Family-Based Treatment Association indicate that a central focus of training for treatment foster caregivers is parent management training (PMT; Kazdin, 1997; Patterson, 1976, 1982; Patterson, Chamberlain, and Reid, 1982). Based on principles of social learning theory and influenced by both B. F. Skinner's operant conditioning theories and Patterson's coercive family process framework, PMT coaches parents in strategies designed to increase prosocial behavior and decrease deviant or inappropriate behaviors. The ability of foster caregivers to effectively manage child behavior is central to maintaining placements (Brown and Bednar, 2006; James, 2004), and increased levels of problem behavior have been shown to relate directly to placement failure (Chamberlain, Price, Reid, Landsverk, Fisher, and Stoolmiller, 2006). Thus, effective training for foster parents in methods that decrease problem behavior is integral in not only preventing placement failure but also reducing the negative impact of subsequent placement instability as discussed above. Scores of studies have been conducted on the effectiveness of PMT for reducing problematic behaviors, and the evidence is extremely robust (see meta-analyses, Eyeburg, Nelson, and Boogs, 2008; Kaminksi, Valle, Filene, and Boyle, 2008; Lundahl, Nimer, and Parsons, 2006; Lundahl, Risser, and Lovejoy, 2006; Maughn, Christiansen, Jenson, Olympia, and Clark, 2005; Serketich and Dumas, 1996; Weisz, Weiss, Han, Granger, and Morton, 1995).

Multidimensional Treatment Foster Care (MTFC). Developed at the Oregon Social Learning Center, MTFC (Chamberlain and Reid, 1991, 1998; Fisher and Chamberlain, 2000) is an evidence-based intervention model that provides comprehensive and intensive support for foster children ages 3–18. The program is designed to be an alternative to regular foster care, residential or group treatment, and incarceration for children with chronic behavior problems. Program staff work across multiple settings (i.e., home, school, and community) and with numerous adjunct providers (i.e., caseworkers, teachers, parole officers, psychiatrists, and attorneys) to increase prosocial behaviors, establish structure in daily routines, maintain high levels of supervision, implement consistent therapeutic limits for problem behavior, and increase placement stability. MTFC foster caregivers participate in a 20-hour preservice training focused on the principles of behavior change rooted in social learning theory and PMT (Patterson, 1976, 1982; Patterson et al., 1982). Given the chronicity and frequency of behavior problems among children living in MTFC homes, foster caregivers maintain contact with clinical staff and other foster caregivers for ongoing training and support needs several times a week, and 24/7 on-call support is provided.

Keeping Foster and Kin Parents Trained and Supported (KEEP). With its roots in the MTFC model of foster caregiver training, the KEEP program was developed as an intervention for regular foster and kinship caregivers of children ages 5–11 (Chamberlain, Moreland, and Reid, 1992; Price, Chamberlain, Landsverk, and Reid, 2009). Building on the core component of foster caregiver training and support, KEEP families participate in a 16-week group training that emphasizes use of positive reinforcement, effective discipline practices, and monitoring. Unlike MTFC, KEEP families do not receive intensive case management or on-call support. Findings indicate that the intervention is effective in reducing behavior problems as a result of caregiver training and increases the likelihood of a successful reunification with families of origin (Price et al., 2009).

APPLICATIONS OF MINDFULNESS-ORIENTED THERAPIES IN RESEARCH AND PRACTICE

Defining the Construct

In recent years, research on mindfulness and its application in the field of mental health has increased exponentially. As researchers and clinicians gain interest, conceptualizations of the mindfulness construct abound. How can the application of mindfulness-oriented therapies improve outcomes for foster children and their caregivers? In order to begin this discussion, a clear definition of mindfulness is warranted. Mindfulness primarily refers to one's perception of stimuli and evaluation thereof.

Although mindfulness in clinical practice has been secularized, its roots in Buddhist and yogic culture lend insight to its definition as a construct. A Buddhist philosopher and scholar wrote that mindfulness can be conceptualized as follows:

> ...pure attentiveness, an alert, impartial function of mind that simply notes whatever appears by way of the senses of sight, hearing, smell, taste, touch, and mind itself. Mindfulness does not cogitate, judge, or interpret; it only observes, neutrally and without commentary, the actual character of an object or phenomenon. (Nyanasobhano, 1998, pp. 16–17)

In a broad definition, Kabat-Zinn (1994) wrote that mindfulness can be defined as "paying attention in a particular way: on purpose, in the present moment, and nonjudgmentally." (p. 4).

Baer (2003) wrote that "mindfulness is the nonjudgmental observation of the ongoing stream of internal and external stimuli as they arise." (p. 125). As one practices mindfulness, phenomenon that enter one's awareness (e.g., thoughts, sensations, and emotions) are observed carefully but not evaluated in a dualistic fashion as good or bad, important or trivial, or true or false (Marlatt and Kristeller, 1999). What is salient across definitions is the notion of the acceptance of what is, being fully present and attentive to the moment while refraining from emotional or evaluative reaction.

Similarities and Clarification

Mindfulness must be distinguished from other similar constructs. The term "attention training" has been used as both a synonym to mindfulness as well as its own practice. While mindfulness does entail the application of selectively attending to a presenting stimulus, we pose that as, it is described primarily in the literature, attention training as a term subsumes this action in its entirety excluding the nonevaluative acceptance component of mindfulness. For application on a variety of mental health targets, attention training primarily addresses ruminative thinking patterns. Wells (1990), for example, developed an attention training technique that is reported to result in flexible control over attention which fosters a shift in information processing from internal cues to external cues, activating a metacognitive action, and subsequently decreasing symptoms of depression, anxiety, social phobia, panic disorder, and hypochondriasis (Papageorgiou and Wells, 1998, 2000; Wells, 1990, 2000; Wells, White, and Carter, 1997). Amir and colleagues developed an attention modification program using linguistic probes or faces displayed on a computer screen, and participants were prompted to shift their attention to neutral cues. Results indicated symptom reduction in attentional bias toward threat for participants with Generalized Anxiety Disorder (Amir, Beard, Burns, and Bomyea, 2009) and social phobia (Amir, Beard, Taylor, et al., 2009). Similarly, Schmidt, Richey, Buckner, and Timpano (2009) used attention training techniques to successfully ameliorate symptoms of social anxiety disorder compared to a control group and gains were maintained at follow-up.

Mindfulness also should be distinguished from basic relaxation. While relaxation is often a byproduct of practicing mindfulness and many mindfulness training protocols include a relaxation component, the purpose of a relaxation exercise is to decrease arousal and stress, whereas the purpose of mindfulness is to cultivate a nonjudgmental awareness: two distinctly different targets. In some instances, mindfulness might actually preclude relaxation; the observer may be orienting to tension, racing thoughts, or irritation, all of which may be incompatible with relaxation.

Lastly, important distinctions need be made between mindfulness and meditation. "Meditation" is broadly defined and encompasses a wide variety of techniques which may or may not include mindfulness. In fact, some forms of meditation run counter to mindfulness entirely as they entail focusing attention on a single stimulus (e.g., word or mantra) and exclude observance of other present moment conditions, whereas mindfulness encourages absolute attention of the moment-to-moment flow of experiences, both internal and external.

Given these distinctions, mindfulness is set apart as a state of focused awareness to the present moment without attachment or qualification; it is a state of dispassionate observance and acceptance of what is.

Current Applications of Mindfulness

Over the last two decades, numerous mindfulness training interventions and clinical applications have emerged. Mindfulness-Based Stress Reduction (MBSR; Kabat-Zinn, 1990) is among the most well-known and has been used to address a host of physical and psychological maladies. MBSR is a multicomponent training program delivered primarily in groups over several weeks and teaches participants to practice mindfulness while mentally scanning the body during seated meditation with focus on breathing and while practicing simple hatha yoga postures.

Mindfulness-Based Cognitive Therapy (MBCT; Teasdale, Segal, and Williams, 1995) is a manualized 8-week group intervention based largely on Kabat-Zinn's MBSR protocol. The primary target of MBCT is to prevent the relapse of depression by practicing detachment from one's thoughts (e.g., "I am not my thoughts"). This decentered thinking is thought to interrupt a potential cascade of ruminative thoughts that can escalate into a more significant depressive episode.

Singh, Wahler, Adkins, and Myers (2003) initially developed a mindfulness training curriculum, Soles of the Feet, for a young man with mental retardation for the purpose of decreasing aggression. Since that initial study, numerous other single subject multiple baseline studies have been conducted using this curriculum with adolescents with conduct disorder (Singh et al., 2007a) and aggressive individuals with severe mental illness (Singh et al., 2007b). The training consists of teaching the individual to focus their attention onto the soles of their feet (a neutral location), practicing mindfulness of this area until their arousal level decreases. Singh and colleagues have also trained parents of children with autism engaging in disruptive and self-injurious behavior (Singh et al., 2006) and parents of children with developmental disabilities (Singh et al., 2007c) in mindfulness practices, although the intervention components of these studies are less clearly articulated.

Integrative Body–Mind Training (IBMT) is another mindfulness-based technique. Developed in the 1990s, its effects have been studied in China since 1995. IBMT achieves the desired state by first giving a brief instructional period on the method called an "initial mind setting" for the purpose of preparing the individual to engage fully in the training. The IBMT method stresses no effort to control thoughts, but instead a state of restful alertness that allows a high degree of awareness (mindfulness) of body, breathing, and the recorded training instructions. The goal is a balanced state of relaxation with focused attention. Thought control is achieved gradually through the aid of a coach who guides posture and relaxation to cultivate a state of body–mind harmony. The purpose of the coach is to minimize the trainee's internal struggle to control thoughts in accordance with instruction. Based on the results from hundreds of adults and children ranging from 4 to 90 years old in China, IBMT has demonstrated improvements in emotional and cognitive performance as well as social behavior (Tang, 2009; Tang et al., 2007, 2009).

In addition to the interventions discussed above, many well-researched and highly utilized therapies include components of mindfulness. Acceptance and Commitment Therapy (Hayes, Strosahl, and Wilson, 1999) is based in behavior analytic principles. While its treatment methods are not described as mindfulness practices per se, they are functionally comparable: namely, the nonjudgmental observation of thoughts and emotions as they arise. In contrast, Dialectical Behavior Therapy (Linehan, 1993) names mindfulness as a core component of its methodology. Principally, mindfulness is practiced as a method to increase acceptance and tolerate distress when it occurs.

Outcomes of Mindfulness Training Studies

The aforementioned treatment models do not comprise an exhaustive list of clinical applications of mindfulness; rather, they represent some of the most notable and well-researched interventions. Intervention studies examining the outcomes of mindfulness training programs (e.g., MBSR and MBCT) and mindfulness-oriented interventions indicate that these methods can be effective for treatment of a variety of disorders. Although critiques have been made regarding methodology (e.g., small sample sizes, lack of control group, and lack of fidelity monitoring), effect sizes for mindfulness interventions have been noted in the medium-to-large range, with the greatest effect for those participants dealing with anxiety and depression problems. In a meta-analysis of mindfulness training intervention studies, Baer (2003) reported that effect sizes at posttreatment ranged from 0.15 to 1.65, with an average weighted mean of 0.59. These were maintained at follow-up. In addition, participants have reported a great deal of satisfaction with the interventions and attribute changes in symptoms to the training they received.

Anxiety and Depression

Mindfulness training has been shown to effectively reduce symptoms of depression (Biegel, Brown, Shapiro, and Schubert, 2009; Kumar, Feldman, and Hayes, 2008; Teasdale et al., 1995; Tang, 2009) and anxiety (Kabat-Zinn et al., 1992; Miller et al., 1995; Vietin and Astin, 2008; Weinstein, Brown, and Ryan, 2009). The mechanisms underlying the effectiveness of mindfulness training in reducing symptomotology are hypothesized to be the training of attention in order to decrease ruminative thinking and the promotion of acceptance (Coffey and Hartman, 2008; Teasdale et al., 1995), which leads to a decrease in avoidance behaviors (Weinstein et al., 2009). The decrease in avoidance behaviors has important implications for anxiety. In one study, individuals high on avoidance measures experienced greater panic symptoms compared to peers lower on avoidance (Karekla, Forsyth, and Kelly, 2004). Avoidance and suppression has actually been shown to result in increases in intrusive thoughts and intensification of associated negative emotions (Davies and Clark, 1998; Wegner and Zanakos, 1994), whereas more active coping (e.g., dealing directly with a stressful situation) and acceptance results in greater adaptation and overall well-being (Weinstein et al., 2009).

Stress and Well-Being

Mindfulness has been shown to have strong associations with stress and overall well-being. Weinstein and colleagues (2009) reported that mindful individuals appraised potentially stressful experiences as more benign than individuals lower in mindfulness and reported less frequent use of avoidant coping strategies. Brown and Ryan (2003) found that mindful individuals experience lower levels of stress and mood disturbance. Tang and colleagues (2007) reported finding significant decreases in stress-related cortisol levels after a short-term mindfulness meditation training.

Improvements in well-being on both physical and mental health dimensions for those dealing with chronic illness have been noted widely. Studies have focused primiarily on the use of MBSR as a primary or adjunct therapy for a number of chronic medical conditions (e.g., chronic pain, fibromyalgia, heart disease, obesity, cancer, and psoriasis; Goldenberg et al., 1994; Kabat-Zinn, Lipworth, and Burney, 1985; Kabat-Zinn, Lipworth, Burney, and Sellars, 1986; Kaplan, Goldenberg, and Galvin-Nadeau, 1993; Ledesma and Kumano, 2009; Lush, Salmon, Floyd, Studts, Weissbecker, and Sephton, 2009). In a meta-analysis examining the effect of MBSR on stress reduction and health benefits, Grossman, Niemann, Schmidt, and Walach (2004) reported moderate effect sizes on both mental and physical health outcomes indicating improvements in quality of life, medical symptoms, and pain. This is likely due in part to the significant effect mindfulness training has on stress, thereby mediating stress-related correlates.

Attention

Discussion of how mindfulness mediates attentional focus and its effects on depression and anxiety are discussed above. Direct impact on attention as it pertains to performance, ADHD symptomotology, and basic orienting has also been demonstrated in the literature. Tang and colleagues (2007) found that even short-term training (100 minutes across 5 days) in IBMT led to better performance in conflict monitoring on the Attention Network Test. Similarly, Jha, Krompinger, and Baime (2007) found that functioning across all three attention networks (alerting, orienting, and conflict monitoring) improved after mindfulness training. Even in the presence of emotional interference, mindfulness meditation training resulted in greater attention control as compared to relaxation training (Ortner, Kilner, and Zelazo, 2007). Sustained attention has also been exhibited with greater proficiency among mindful individuals compared with controls (Schmertz, Anderson, and Robins, 2009; Valentine and Sweet, 1999). Interestingly, very little research on mindfulness applications for individuals with ADHD has been conducted. In one feasibility study, the majority of adult and adolescent participants with ADHD completed the training; although behavioral improvements were noted at posttest, the lack of randomization and a control group indicated the need for a more methodologically rigorous examination (Zylowska et al., 2007).

Self-Regulation

Mindfulness is not typically applied as an intervention to regulate mood and behavior per se but rather to observe emotions or thoughts in a nonjudgmental, nonreactive manner. This can result in a decrease in physiological arousal as the individual turns his/her attention to a neutral posture in response to a potentially provoking incident. This is a central construct behind emotion regulation and has neurophysiological implications as well. After administering fMRIs during an affect labeling task, Creswell and colleagues (2007) found that individuals with high levels of mindfulness exhibited increased prefrontal cortex activation and decreased amygdala activity lending credence to this relationship. Tang and colleagues (2009) observed increased activation in ventral anterior cingulate cortex, the self-regulation center in the brain (Posner et al., 2007), after only 5 days of IBMT in comparison to 5 days of relaxation training.

As discussed above, the conflict monitoring component of attention (e.g., executive control) is central to self-regulation, and we have discussed how mindfulness training impacts this network. Another theory as to how mindfulness influences self-regulation is seen in self-determination theory (Ryan and Deci, 2000), which posits that open awareness, as is demonstrated in mindfulness, may be particularly facilitative in one's ability to select behavioral responses congruent to one's interest, values, or needs. Brown and Ryan (2003) found that mindfulness was actually predictive of self-regulation in day-to-day activities. In one study with adolescents demonstrating externalizing behavior problems, mindfulness training resulted in a significant decrease of both self-reported and parent-reported complaints of externalizing behaviors (Bogels, Hoogstad, van Dun, de Schutter, and Restifo, 2008).

The findings from another study indicated an inverse relationship between mindfulness and aggression and hostile attribution bias and that, after mindfulness training, individuals responded to provocation with lower levels of aggression and hostile attribution bias than control groups (Heppner et al., 2008).

Children and Adolescents

Applications for youth have been severely understudied to date. The mean age range of participants in published mindfulness studies has been 38–50 years. Of the few existing studies, only a handful were methodologically sound; thus, implications for treatment have been somewhat speculative. Semple, Lee, and Miller (2006) explained that, although the results from adult studies have been promising, the research with children and adolescents "has barely begun" (p. 164). The bulk of the studies with youth have involved nonclinical populations, small sample feasibility studies, case studies, or measuring outcomes anecdotally or without the use of validated instruments (Thompson and Gauntlett-Gilbert, 2008). Complicating matters further, there is only one mindfulness measure validated for use with children to date, the Child and Adolescent Mindfulness Measure (Greco, Dew, and Baer, 2005).

It is important to note, however, that the lack of a substantial body of rigorous research with youth does not mean that mindfulness training in this population is infeasible or without promise. A small number of studies have been conducted, indicating that not only can mindfulness be trained in children and adolescents but that training may have important implications for health and well-being. Schoeberlein and Koffler (2005) worked with the Garrison Institute to examine contemplative programs with children ages 5–18 throughout the United States. They found that, during the 2004–2005 school year, over 20 school- and community-based programs prioritizing mindfulness, attention training, emotional balance, and well-being were being implemented, indicating high feasibility for instructing children and adolescents in these methods. Although none of these programs reported empirical data, the report indicated general increases in self-awareness, self-reflection, emotional intelligence, and social skills. Other studies with children and adolescents, while not all methodologically rigorous, report training participants' ranging from 4–19 years old in mindfulness techniques (Biegel et al., 2009; Lee, Semple, Rosa, and Miller, 2008; Miller, Wyman, Huppert, Glassman, and Rathaus, 2000; Napoli, Krech, and Holley, 2005; Ott, 2002; Semple et al., 2006; Semple, Reid, and Miller, 2005; Singh et al., 2007a; Tang, 2005, 2007; Wall, 2005). Training methods with youth necessitate developmental considerations as attention, self-regulatory, cognitive, linguistic, and interpersonal abilities vary distinctly from adults and throughout stages of childhood.

Potential Mindfulness Applications in Foster Care

Foster Caregivers and Biological Parents

Given the prior discussion regarding the intensive needs of foster children, it bears repeating that providing responsive, nurturing care for these children can be extraordinarily difficult. In fact, clinical support for foster caregivers who serve these children has been found to be integral to maintaining placement stability and decreasing parenting stress (Fisher and Stoolmiller, 2008). Foster caregiver stress has also been shown to have a negative association on child physiological functioning (Fisher and Stoolmiller, 2008). Many foster parents of children with chronic emotional and behavioral problems describe living in a constant state of triage, which ultimately compromises their effectiveness in parenting and maintaining a therapeutic approach. Even when one has the knowledge and training needed to be effective, stress and overwhelm can dramatically interfere with the ability to access that knowledge and respond in accordance with a more goal-directed approach.

To further complicate matters, foster children often experience the early parent–child relationship as chronically rejection oriented and reactive. As they enter foster care, very little may appear familiar, particularly in regard to the new parent–child framework. This results in a rather distinct dynamic. The foster child must take time to learn the norms and expectations of the foster family as well as how to appropriately initiate interactions and how to respond. During the process, they often engage in the more familiar rejection-oriented and reactive parent–child dynamic, pulling for what is familiar. In addition to what is often an already substantial constellation of emotional and behavioral needs, the best intentions of the foster caregiver to support the child is undercut by the elicitation of antagonistic exchanges. Reactivity on the part of the foster caregiver can serve to undermine therapeutic progress for the child. Given this, applications for mindfulness training for foster caregivers could result in (1) increases in goal-directed parenting, (2) improved utilization of evidence-based therapeutic parenting practices as a result of improved self-regulation and decreased arousal, (3) reductions in stress, and (4) improved well-being, all of which lead to greater placement stability and more positive child outcomes.

Similarly, biological parents may benefit from mindfulness training. Fisher, Burraston, and Pears (2005) found that a significant number of permanent placements failed less than 1 year after reunification. Although the reasons for these failures still need to be fully explicated, it is often the case that, as the child begins to stabilize in the home, services and supports are likely to end. Parents may not have the long-term emotional resources to cope with the stressors of parenting a high-needs child; consequently, placements may deteriorate. The benefit of mindfulness training for these families may also serve to buffer these numerous risk factors.

Foster Children

Training foster children in mindfulness strategies has the potential to make a unique contribution to their treatment. We have highlighted the impact that mindfulness has on attentional focus, executive functioning, self-regulation, depression, and anxiety, all of which are well-documented needs among foster children. Important social correlates are targets for these interventions as well, namely hostile attribution bias, emotion regulation, and enhanced self-awareness. In addition, mindfulness supports coping with stressors and enhances overall well-being, which are important protective factors with the potential of increasing resilience in the face of adversity. Finally, mindfulness practices have been shown to support healthy neurophysiological functioning, which fosters continued adaptation to environmental demands. Outcomes from mindfulness training may extend to academic environments as well and warrant exploration in this setting given the poor academic functioning exhibited in this population.

Follette, Palm, and Pearson (2006) posed that integrating mindfulness techniques into treatment for trauma may be particularly effective at supporting cognitive flexibility, focusing on the present, and supporting acceptance. In fact, in one study, mindfulness factors (i.e., accepting without judgment and acting with awareness) were predictive of PTSD symptoms in a sample of 239 adults who reported exposure to trauma but did not meet criteria for PTSD (Vujanovic, Youngwirth, Johnson, and Zvolensky, 2009). This is particularly salient as many foster children evidence posttraumatic symptomotology without a formal Axis I diagnosis.

FUTURE DIRECTIONS

The study of mindfulness training and mindfulness-oriented interventions is growing exponentially as scientists and clinicians gain interest. There are a number of exciting domains yet to explore. With regard to children and adolescents, feasibility and modalities for training, mechanisms of action, impact of training on neurophysiological functioning, methods for generalization of skills, and measurement of mindfulness outcomes are just a few of the domains waiting to be explored in greater depth. As of yet, research on training mindfulness with foster children and their caregivers has yet to be conducted, but the implications of this work are exciting from both a basic science and clinical perspectives. Additionally, the feasibility and impact of mindfulness training on foster children with concurrent developmental disabilities will be an promising area to explore.

Mindfulness training has the potential to increase the effectiveness of already robust methodologies by targeting the intrapersonal obstacles to effective implementation of methods. Three-prong studies that include a treatment group, treatment plus mindfulness, and matched controls may serve to illuminate the function of these obstacles and highlight strategies for eliminating them.

Longitudinal follow-up after mindfulness training for foster children may also highlight the potential for mindfulness to serve as a protective factor, over time increasing favorable outcomes compared to children lower in mindfulness abilities. In fact, mindfulness studies have the potential to make a meaningful contribution to the study of resilience and risk prevention as it may be an important axis point for a number of critical risk factors. Additionally, longitudinal studies examining time-limited mindfulness training interventions, interventions with generalization protocols, interventions with and without booster sessions, caregiver involvement and training, and training across various ages and stages may illuminate critical windows and modalities for maximally beneficial outcomes.

In short, we are at the beginning stages of an exciting inquiry process examining an age-old technique. With many avenues to explore, mindfulness training and its potential to impact such high-risk populations as those described here will no doubt engage researchers and clinicians for many years to come.

The strength and meaning of this endeavor, however, will be in direct proportion to the rigors of methodology we observe during this inquiry. Indeed, mindfulness presents a ripe opportunity to marry the best of science and practice.

REFERENCES

Achenbach, T. M. (1991). Manual for the Child Behavior Checklist/4-18 and 1991 Profile. Burlington: University of Vermont.

Ackerman, B. P., Brown, E. and Izard, C. E. (2003). Continuity and change in levels of externalizing behavior in school of children from economically disadvantaged families. *Child Development*, 74, 694–709.

Ackerman, B. P., Brown, E., D'Eramo, K. S. and Izard, C. E. (2002). Maternal relationship instability and the school behavior of children from disadvantaged families. *Developmental Psychology*, 38, 694–704.

Ackerman, B. P., Kogos, J., Youngstrom, E., Schoff, K. and Izard, C. (1999). Family instability and the problem behaviors of children from economically disadvantaged families. *Developmental Psychology*, 35, 258–268.

Ackerman, P. T., Newton, J. E. O., McPherson, W. B., Jones, J. G. and Dykman, R. A. (1998). Prevalence of post traumatic stress disorder and other psychiatric diagnoses in three groups of abused children (sexual, physical, and both). *Child Abuse and Neglect*, 22, 759–774.

Albano, A. M. and Kendall, P. C. (2002). Cognitive behavioral therapy for children and adolescents with anxiety disorders: Clinical research advances. *International Review of Psychiatry*, 14, 129–134.

Amir, N., Beard, C., Burns, M. and Bomyea, J. (2009). Attention modification program in individuals with generalized anxiety disorder. *Journal of Abnormal Psychology*, 118, 28–33.

Amir, N., Beard, C., Taylor, C. T., Klumpp, H., Elias, J., Burns, M. and Chen, X. (2009). Attention training in individuals with generalized social phobia: A randomized control trial. *Journal of Consulting and Clinical Psychology*, 77, 961–973.

Asarnow, J. R., Jaycox, L. H. and Tompson, M. C. (2001). Depression in youth: psychosocial interventions. *Journal of Clinical Child Psychology*, 30, 33–47.

Baer, R. A. (2003). Mindfulness training as a clinical intervention: a conceptual and empirical review. *Clinical Psychology: Science and Practice, 10, 125*–143.

Baer, R. A. and Neitzel, M. T. (1991). Cognitive and behavioral treatment of impulsivity in children: A meta-analytic review of the outcome literature. *Journal of Clinical Child Psychology*, 20, 400–412.

Barbell, L. (1997). Foster care today: A briefing paper. Washington, DC: Child Welfare League of America.

Barbell, K. and Freundlich, M. (2001). Foster care today. Washington, DC: Casey Family Programs.

Bar-Haim, Y., Lamy, D., Pergamin, L., Bakermans-Kranenburg, M. J. and van IJzendoorn, M. H. (2007). Threat-related attentional bias in anxious and nonanxious individuals: A meta-analytic study. *Psychological Bulletin*, 133, 1–12.

Barkley, R. A. (1997). Behavioral inhibition, sustained attention, and executive functions: Constructing a unifying theory of ADHD. *Psychological Bulletin, 121, 65–94.*

Benbenishty, R. and Oyserman, D. (1995). Children in foster care: Their present situation and plans for their future. *International Social Work, 38*, 117–131.

Bendixen, M., Muus, K. M. and Schei, B. (1994). The impact of child sexual abuse – a study of a random sample of Norwegian students. *Child Abuse and Neglect*, 18, 837–847.

Benton, A. (1991). Prefrontal injury and behavior in children. *Developmental Neuropsychology, 7*, 275–281.

Biegel, G. M., Brown, K. W., Shapiro, S. L. and Schubert, C. M. (2009). Mindfulness-based stress reduction for the treatment of adolescent psychiatric outpatients: A randomized clinical trial. *Journal of Consulting and Clinical Psychology*, 77, 855–866.

Birch, S. H. and Ladd, G. W. (1998). Children's interpersonal behaviors and the teacher-child relationship. *Developmental Psychology*, 34, 934–946.

Bogels, S., Hoogstad, B., van Dun, L., de Schutter, S. and Restifo, K. (2008). Mindfulness training for adolescents with externalizing disorders and their parents. *Behavioural and Cognitive Psychotherapy*, 36, 193–209.

Bolger, K. E. and Patterson, C. J. (2003). Sequelae of child maltreatment: Vulnerability and resilience. In S. S. Luthar (Ed.), Resilience and Vulnerability: Adaptation in the Context of Childhood Adversities (156–181). New York, NY: Cambridge University.

Bradley, S. J. (2000). Affect regulation and the development of psychopathology. New York: Guilford.

Braswell, L. and Kendall, P. C. (2003). Cognitive-behavioral therapy with youth. In Dobson, K. S. (Ed.), Handbook of cognitive behavioral therapies (246–294). New York: Guilford.

Brown, J. D. and Bednar, L. M. (2006). Foster parent perceptions of placement breakdown. *Children and Youth Services Review*, 28, 1497–1511.

Brown, K. W. and Ryan, R. M. (2003). The benefits of being present: Mindfulness and its role in psychological well-being. *Journal of Personality and Social Psychology*, 84, 822–848.

Bruce, J., Davis, E. P. and Gunnar, M. R. (2002). Individual differences in children's cortisol response to the beginning of a new school year. *Psychoneuroendocrinology*, 27, 635–650.

Celano M. and Rothbaum, B. O. (2002). Psychotherapeutic approaches with survivors of childhood trauma. *Seminars in Clinical Neuropsychiatry*, 7, 120–128.

Chamberlain, P. (1994). Family connections: A treatment foster care model for adolescents with delinquency. Eugene, OR: Castalia Publishing.

Chamberlain, P. (2002). Treatment foster care. In B. Burns, and K. Hoagwood (Eds.), Community treatment for youth: Evidence-based interventions for severe emotional and behavioral disorders (pp. 117–138). New York: Oxford University.

Chamberlain, P., Moreland, S. and Reid, K. (1992). Enhanced services and stipends for foster parents: Effects on retention rates and outcomes for children. *Child Welfare*, 71, 387–401.

Chamberlain, P., Price, J. M., Reid, J. B., Landsverk, J., Fisher, P. A. and Stoolmiller, M. (2006). Who disrupts from placement in foster and kinship care? *Child Abuse and Neglect*, 30, 409–424.

Chamberlain, P. and Reid, J. B. (1991). Using a specialized foster care treatment model for children and adolescents leaving the state mental hospital. *Journal of Community Psychology*, 19, 266–276.

Chamberlain, P. and Reid, J. (1998). Comparison of two community alternatives to incarceration for chronic juvenile offenders. *Journal of Consulting and Clinical Psychology, 6, 624–633.*

Chernoff, R., Combs-Orme, T., Risley-Curtis, C. and Heiser, A. (1994). Assessing the health status of children entering foster care. *Pediatrics*, 93, 594–601.

Cicchetti, D., Ackerman, B. P. and Izard, C. E. (1995). Emotions and emotion regulation in developmental psychopathology. *Development and Psychopathology*, 7, 1–10.

Cicchetti, D. and Toth, S. (1995). Child maltreatment and attachment organization: Implications for intervention. In S., Goldberg, R. Muir, and J. Kerr, (Eds.), Attachment theory: Social, developmental, and clinical perspectives (pp. 279–308). London: The Analytical Press.

Clausen, J. M., Landsverk, J., Ganger, W., Chadwick, D. and Litrownik, A. (1998). Mental health problems of children in foster care. *Journal of Child and Family Studies*, 7, 283–296.

Coffey, K. and Hartman, M. (2008). Mechanisms of action in the inverse relationship between mindfulness and psychological distress. *Complementary Health Practice Review*, 13, 79–91.

Cohen, J. A., Deblinger, E., Mannarino, A. P. and Steer, R. (2004). A multi-site randomized controlled trial for sexually abused children with PTSD symptoms. *Journal of the American Academy of Child and Adolescent Psychiatry*, 43, 393–402.

Cohen, J. A. and Mannarino, A. P. (2004). Treatment of childhood traumatic grief. *Journal of Clinical Child and Adolescent Psychology*, 33, 820–832.

Cohen, J. A. and Mannarino, A. P. (2008). Trauma-focused cognitive behavioural therapy for children and parents. *Child and Adolescent Mental Health*, 13, 158–162.

Cohen, J. A., Mannarino, A. P., Perel, J. M. and Staron, V. (2007). A pilot randomized controlled trial of combined trauma-focused CBT and sertraline for childhood PTSD symptoms. *Journal of the American Academy of Child and Adolescent Psychiatry*, 46, 811–819.

Compas, B. E. and Oppedisano, G. (2000). *Mixed anxiety/ depression in childhood and adolescence*. In A. J., Sameroff, M. Lewis, and S. M. Miller, (Eds), Handbook of Developmental Psychopathology (pp. 531–548). New York: Klewer Academic/Plenum Publishers.

Creswell, J. D., Way. B. M., Eisenberger, N. I. and Lieberman, M. D. (2007). Neural correlates of dispositional mindfulness during affect labeling. *Psychosomatic Medicine*, 69, 560–565.

Davidson, R. J. (2000). Affective style, psychopathology, and resilience: Brain mechanisms and plasticity. *American Psychologist*, 55, 1196–1214.

Davies, M. I. and Clark, D. M. (1998). Thought suppression produces rebound effect with analogue post-traumatic intrusions. *Behavioral Research and Therapy*, 36, 571–582.

Denham, S. A., Blair, K. A., DeMulder, E., Levitas, J., Sawyer, K. and Auerbach-Major, S., et al. (2003). Preschool emotional competence: Pathway to social competence. *Child Development*, 74, 238–256.

Dorsey, S., Farmer, E. M. Z., Barth, R. P., Greene, K. M., Reid, J. and Landsverk, J. (2008). Current status and evidence base of training for foster and treatment foster parents. *Children and Youth Services Review*, 30, 1403–1416.

Dubowitz, H. (1990). The physical and mental health and educational status of children placed with relatives: Final report. Baltimore, MD: Department of Pediatrics, School of Medicine. University of Maryland.

Eckenrode, J., Laird, M. and Doris, J. (1993). School performance and disciplinary problems among abused and neglected children. *Developmental Psychology*, 29, 53–62.

Eisenberg, N., Sadovsky, A., Spinrad, T. L., Fabes, R. A., Losoya, S. H. and Valiente, C., et al. (2005). The relations of problem behavior status to children's negative emotionality, effortful control, and impulsivity: Concurrent relations and prediction of change. *Developmental Psychology*, 41, 193–211.

Eisenberg, N. and Spinrad, T. L. (2004). Emotion-related regulation: Sharpening the definition. *Child Development*, 75, 334–339.

English, A. and Grasso, K. (1999). The Foster Care Independence Act of 1999: Enhancing youth access to health care. *Clearinghouse Review/Journal of Poverty Law and Policy*, 224, 217–32.

Eyeburg, S. M., Nelson, M. M. and Boggs, S. R. (2008). Evidence-based psychosocial treatments for children and adolescents with disruptive behavior. *Journal of Clinical Child and Adolescent Psychiatry*, 37, 215–237.

Feather, J. and Ronan, K. R. (2006). Trauma-focused Cognitive Behavioral Therapy for abused children with Post-traumatic Stress Disorder: A pilot study. *New Zealand Journal of Psychology*, 35, 132–145.

Fisher, P. A., Burraston, B. and Pears, K. C. (2005). The Early Intervention Foster Care Program: Permanent placement outcomes from a randomized trial. *Child Maltreatment*, 10, 61–71.

Fisher, P. A. and Chamberlain, P. (2000). Multidimensional treatment foster care: A program for intensive parenting, family support, and skill building. *Journal of Emotional and Behavioral Disorders*, 8, 155–164.

Fisher, P. A. and Stoolmiller, M. (2008). Intervention effects on foster parent stress: Associations with child cortisol levels. *Development and Psychopathology*, 20(3), 1003–1021.

Follette, V., Palm, K. M. and Pearson, A. N. (2006). Mindfulness and trauma: Implications for treatment. *Journal of Rational Emotive and Cognitive-Behavior Therapy*, 24, 45–61.

Garon, N., Bryson, S. E. and Smith, I. M. (2008). Executive function in preschoolers: A review using an integrative framework. *Psychological Bulletin*, 134, 31–60.

Glisson, C., Bailey J. W. and Post, J. A. (2000). Predicting the time children spend in state custody. *Social Service Review*, 74, 253–280.

Goldenberg, D. L., Kaplan, K. H., Nadeau, M. G., Brodeur, G., Smith, S. and Schmid, G. H. (1994). A controlled study of a stress-reduction cognitive-behavioral treatment program in fibromyalgia. *Journal of Musculoskeletal Pain*, 2, 53–66.

Greco, L. A., Dew, S. E. and Baer, R. (2005). Acceptance, mindfulness, and related processes in childhood: Measurement issues, clinical relevance, and future directions. In S. E. Dew, and R. Baer, (Chairs), Measuring acceptance, mindfulness, and related processes: Empirical findings and clinical applications across child, adolescent, and adult samples. Symposium presented at the Association for Behavior and Cognitive Therapies, Washington, D.C.

Grossman, P., Niemann, L., Schmidt, S. and Walach, H. (2004). Mindfulness-based stress reduction and health benefits: A meta-analysis. *Journal of Psychosomatic Research*, 57, 35–43.

Gunnar, M., Fisher, P. A. and The Early Experience, Stress, and Prevention Network. (2006). Bringing basic research on early experience and stress neurobiology to bear on preventive interventions for neglected and maltreated children. *Development and Psychopathology*, 18, 651–677.

Hayes, S. C., Strosahl, K. and Wilson, K. G. (1999). Acceptance and Commitment Therapy. New York: Guilford.

Hernandez, J. (1992). Eating disorders and sexual abuse among adolescents. Chapel Hill, NC: The University of North Carolina at Chapel Hill. (ERIC Document Reproduction Service No. ED358404).

Heppner, W. L., Kernis, M. H., Lakey, C. E., Campbell, W. K., Goldman, B. M., Davis, P. J. and Cascio, E. V. (2008). Mindfulness as a means of reducing aggressive behavior: Dispositional and situational evidence. *Aggressive Behavior*, 34, 486–496.

Hoagwood, K. E., Radigan, M., Rodriguez, J., Levitt, J. M., Fernandez, D., Foster, J. and with NY State Office of Mental Health (2006). Final Report on the Child and Adolescent Trauma Treatment Consortium (CATS) Project. SAMHSA, Unpublished report.

James, S. (2004). Why do foster care placements disrupt? An investigation of reasons for placement change in foster care. *The Social Service Review*, 78, 601– 626.

Jha, A. P., Krompinger, J. and Baime, M. J. (2007). Mindfulness training modifies subsystems of attention. *Cognitive, Affective, and Behavioral Neuroscience*, 7, 109–119.

Kabat-Zinn, J. (1990). Full catastrophe living: Using the wisdom of your body and mind to face stress, pain, and illness. New York: Delacorte.

Kabat-Zinn, J. (1994). Wherever you go, there you are: Mindfulness meditation in everyday life. New York: Hyperion.

Kabat-Zinn, J., Lipworth, L. and Burney, R. G. (1985). The clinical use of mindfulness meditation for the self-regulation of chronic pain. *Journal of Behavioral Medicine*, 8, 163–190.

Kabat-Zinn, J., Lipworth, L, Burney, R. G. and Sellars, W. (1986). Four year follow-up of a meditation based program for the self-regulation of chronic pain: Treatment outcomes and compliance. *Clinical Journal of Pain*, 2, 159–173.

Kabat-Zinn, J., Massion, M. D., Kristeller, J., Peterson, L. G., Fletcher, K. E. and Pbert, L., et al. (1992). Effectiveness of a meditation-based stress reduction program in the treatment of anxiety disorders. *American Journal of Psychiatry*, 149, 936–943.

Kaminski, J. W., Valle, L. A., Filene, J. H. and Boyle, C. L. (2008). A meta-analytic review of components associated with parent training program effectiveness. *Journal of Abnormal Child Psychology*, 36, 567–589.

Kaplan, K. H., Goldenberg, D. L and Galvin-Nadeau, M. (1993). The impact of a meditation-based stress reduction program on fibromyalgia. *General Hospital Psychiatry*, 15, 284–289.

Karekla, M., Forsyth, J. P. and Kelly, M. M. (2004). Emotional avoidance and panicogenic responding to a biological challenge. *Behavior Therapy*, 35, 725–746.

Kazdin, A. E. (1997). Parent-management training: Evidence, outcomes, and issues. *Journal of the American Academy of Child and Adolescent Psychiatry*, 36, 1349–1356.

Kendall, P. C. (1998). Empirically supported psychosocial therapies. *Journal of Consulting and Clinical Psychology*, 66, 1–3.

Kendall, P. C. (2000). Child and adolescent therapy: Cognitive-behavioral procedures. (2nd ed.). New York: Guilford.

Kendall, J., Dale, G. and Plakitsis, S. (1995). The mental health needs of children entering the Child Welfare system: A guide for case workers. *APSAC Advisor*, 8, 10–13.

Kendall, P. C. and Panichelli-Mindel, S. M. (1995). Cognitive-behavioral treatments. *Journal of Abnormal Child Psychology*, 23, 107–124.

Kiecolt-Glaser, J. K., McGuire, L., Robles, T. F. and Glaser, R. (2002). Emotions, morbidity, and mortality: New perspectives from psychoneuroimmunology. *Annual Review of Psychology*, 53, 83–107.

Kinard, E. M. (1999). Perceived social skills and social competence in maltreated children. *American Journal of Orthopsychiatry*, 69, 465–481.

King, N. J., Tonge, B. J., Mullen, P., Myerson, N., Heyne, D., Rollings, S., Martin, R. and Ollendick, T. H. (2000). Treating sexually abused children with posttraumatic stress symptoms: A randomized clinical trial. *Journal of the American Academy of Child and Adolescent Psychiatry*, 39, 1347–1355.

Kumar, S., Feldman, G. and Hayes, A. (2008). Changes in mindfulness and emotion regulation in an exposure-based cognitive therapy for depression. *Cognitive Therapy and Research*, 32, 734–744.

Ladd, G. W., Birch, S. H. and Buhs, E. S. (1999). Children's social and scholastic lives in kindergarten: Related spheres of influence, *Child Development*, 70, 1373–1400.

Landsverk, J., Davis, I., Ganger, W., Newton, R. and Johnson, I. (1996). Impact of child psychosocial functioning on reunification from out-of-home placement. *Children and Youth Services Review*, 18, 447–462.

Landsverk, J. and Garland, A. F. (1999). Foster care and pathways to mental health services. In P. A., Curtis, G. Dale Jr., and J. C. Kendall, (Eds.). *The foster care crisis (pp.* 193–210). Lincoln, NE: Nebraska Press.

Ledesma, D. and Kumano, H. (2009). Mindfulness-based stress reduction and cancer: A meta-analysis. *Psycho-Oncology*, 18, 571–579.

Lee, J., Semple, R. J., Rosa, D. and Miller, L. (2008). Mindfulness-based cognitive therapy for children: Results of a pilot study. *Journal of Cognitive Psychotherapy: An International Quarterly*, 22, 15–28.

Lewis, E. E., Dozier, M., Ackerman, J. and Sepulveda-Kozakowski, S. (2007). The effect of placement instability on adopted children's inhibitory control abilities and oppositional behavior. *Developmental Psychology*, 43, 1415–1427.

Lewinsohn, P. M., Clarke, G. N., Rohde, P., Hops, H. and Seeley, J. R. (1996). A course in coping: a cognitive-behavioral approach to the treatment of adolescent depression. In E. D. Hibbs, and P. S. Jensen, (Eds.), Child and Adolescent Disorders: Empirically based strategies for clinical practice (pp. 109–135). Washington, DC: American Psychological Association.

Liem, J. H. and Boudewyn, A. C. (1999). Contextualizing the effects of childhood sexual abuse on adult self- and social functioning: An attachment theory perspective. *Child Abuse and Neglect*, 23, 1141–1157.

Linehan, M. M. (1993). Cognitive-behavioral treatment of borderline personality disorder. New York: Guilford.

Lundahl, B. W., Nimer, J. and Parsons, B. (2006). Preventing child abuse: A meta-analysis of parent training programs. *Research on Social Work Practice*, 16, 251–262.

Lundahl, B., Risser, H. J. and Lovejoy, M. C. (2006). A meta-analysis of parent training: Moderators and follow-up effects. *Clinical Psychology Review*, 26, 86–104.

Lush, E., Salmon, P., Floyd, A., Studts, J. L., Weissbecker, I. and Sephton, S. E. (2009). Mindfulness meditation for symptom reduction in fibromyalgia: Psychophysiological correlates. *Journal of Clinical Psychology in Medical Settings*, 16, 200–207.

Marlatt, G. A. and Kristeller, J. L. (1999). Mindfulness and meditation. In W. R. Miller (Ed.), *Integrating spirituality into treatment* (pp. 67–84). Washington, DC: American Psychological Association.

Maughn, D. R., Christiansen, E., Jenson, W. R., Olympia, D. and Clark, E. (2005). Behavioral parent training as a treatment for externalizing behaviors and disruptive behavior disorders: A meta-analysis. *School Psychology Review*, 34, 267–286.

McClelland, M. M., Morrison, F. J. and Holmes, D. L. (2000). Children at risk for early academic problems: The role of learning-related social skills. *Early Childhood Research Quarterly*, 15, 307–329.

McIntyre, A. and Thomas, Y. (1986). Psychological disorders among foster children. Journal of *Clinical Child Psychology*, 15, 297–303.

Mian, M., Marton, P. and LeBaron, D. (1996). The effects of sexual abuse on 3- to 5-year-old girls. *Child Abuse and Neglect*, 20, 731–745.

Miller, J. J., Fletcher, K. and Kabat-Zinn, J. (1995). Three-year follow-up and clinical implications of a mindfulness meditation-based stress reduction intervention in the treatment of anxiety disorders. *General Hospital Psychiatry*, 17, 192–200.

Miller, A. L.,Wyman, S. E., Huppert, J. D., Glassman, S. L. and Rathaus, J. H. (2000). Analysis of behavioural skills utilized by suicidal adolescents receiving dialectical behaviour therapy. *Cognitive and Behavioural Practice*, 7, 183–187.

Mogg, K. and Bradley, B. P. (2005). Attentional bias in generalized anxiety disorder versus depressive disorder. *Cognitive Therapy and Research*, 29, 29–45.

Morris, A. S., Silk, J. S., Steinberg, L., Myers, S. S. and Robinson, L. R. (2007). The role of the family context in the development of emotion regulation. *Social Development*, 16, 361–388.

Napoli, M., Krech, P. R. and Holley, L. C. (2005). Mindfulness training for elementary school students: The Attention Academy. *Journal of Applied School Psychology*, 21, 99–123.

Nelson, W. M. and Finch, A. J. (1996). Keeping your cool: The anger management workbook, Ardmore, PA: Workbook.

Newton, R. R., Litrownik, A. J. and Landsverk, J. A. (2000). Children and youth in foster care: Disentangling the relationship between problem behaviors and number of placements. *Child Abuse and Neglect*, 24, 1363–1374.

Nolen-Hoeksema, S. (2000). The role of rumination in depressive disorders and mixed anxiety/depressive symptoms. *Journal of Abnormal Psychology*, 109, 504–511.

Nyanasobhano, B. (1998). Landscapes of wonder: Discovering Buddhist dharma in the world around us. Boston: Wisdom Publications.

Ollendick, T. H. (1998). Empirically supported treatments for children with phobic and anxiety disorders: Current status. [comment]. *Journal of Clinical Child Psychology*, 27, 234–245.

Ortner, C. N. M., Kilner, S. J. and Zelazo, P. D. (2007). Mindfulness meditation and reduced emotional interference on a cognitive task. *Motivation and Emotion*, 31, 271–283.

Ott, M. J. (2002). Mindfulness meditation in pediatric clinical practice. *Pediatric Nursing*, 28, 487–491.

Papageorgiou, C. and Wells, A. (1998). Effects of attention training on hypochondriasis: a brief case series. *Psychological Medicine*, 28, 193–200.

Papageorgiou, C. and Wells, A. (2000). Treatment of recurrent major depression with attention training. *Cognitive and Behavioral Practice*, 7, 407–413.

Patterson, G. R. (1976). Living with children: New methods for parents and teachers. Champaign, IL: Research Press.

Patterson, G. R. (1982). Coercive family process. Eugene, OR: Castalia.

Patterson, G. R., Chamberlain, P. and Reid, J. B. (1982). A comparative evaluation of parent training procedures. *Behavior Therapy*, 13, 638–650.

Pears, K. A. and Fisher, P. A. (2005). Developmental, cognitive, and neuropsychological functioning in preschool-aged foster children: Associations with prior maltreatment and placement history. *Developmental and Behavioral Pediatrics*, 26, 112–122.

Pennington, B. F. (1997). Dimensions of executive functions in normal and abnormal development. In N. A., Krasnegor, G. R. Lyon, and P. S. Goldman-Rakic, (Eds.), Development of the prefrontal cortex: Evolution, neurobiology, and behavior (265–281). Baltimore, MD: Paul H. Brookes Publishing.

Pilowsky, D. (1995). Psychopathology among children placed in family foster care. *Psychiatric Services*, 46, 906–910.

Posner, M. I. and Dehaene, S. (2004). Attentional networks. *Trends in Neuroscience*, 7, 75–79.

Posner, M. I., Rothbart, M. K., Sheese, B. E. and Tang, Y. (2007). The anterior cingulate gyrus and the mechanism of self-regulation. *Cognitive Affective Behavioral Neuro science*, 7, 391–395.

Price, J. M., Chamberlain, P., Landsverk, J. and Reid, J. (2009). KEEP foster parent training intervention: Model description and effectiveness. *Child and Family Social Work*, 14, 233–242.

Racusin, R., Maerlander, A., Sengupta, A., Straus, M. and Isquith, P. (2003). Executive functions and post-traumatic symptoms in maltreated foster care children. Paper presented at the annual meeting of the American Academy of Child and Adolescent Psychiatry: Miami, FL.

Roeser, R. W. and Eccles, J. S. (2000). Schooling and Mental Health. In A. J., Sameroff, M. Lewis, and S. M. Miller, (Eds), *Handbook of Developmental Psychopathology* (135–156). New York: Klewer Academic/Plenum Publishers.

Rogosch, F. A. and Cicchetti, D. (1994). Illustrating the interface of family and peer relations through the study of child maltreatment, *Social Development*, 3, 291–308.

Rothbart, M. K. and Bates, J. E. (2006). Temperament. In N. Eisenberg, W. Damon, R. M. Lerner (Eds.), Handbook of child psychology: Vol. 3, Social, emotional, and personality development (6th ed., pp. 99–166). Hoboken, NJ: John Wiley and Sons Inc.

Rotheram-Borus, M. J., Piacentini, J., Miller, S., Graae, F. and Castro-Blanco, D. (1994). Brief cognitive-behavioral treatment for adolescent suicide attempters and their families. *Journal of the American Academy of Child and Adolescent Psychiatry*, 33, 508–517.

Rowe, E. and Eckenrode, J. (1999). The timing of academic difficulties among maltreated and nonmaltreated children. *Child Abuse and Neglect*, 23, 813–832.

Roy, P., Rutter, M. and Pickles, A. (2000). Institutional care: Risk from family background or pattern of rearing? *Journal of Child Psychology and Psychiatry*, 41, 139–149.

Rueda, M. R., Posner, M. I. and Rothbart, M. K. (2005). The development of executive attention: Contributions to the emergence of self-regulation. *Developmental Neuropsychology*, 28, 573–594.

Ryan, R. M. and Deci, E. L. (2000). Self-determination theory and the facilitation of intrinsic motivation, social development, and well-being. *American Psychologist*, 55, 68–78.

Rydell, A. M., Berlin, L. and Bohlin, G. (2003). Emotionality, emotion regulation and adaptation among 5- and 8-year-old children. *Emotion*, 3, 30–47.

Salovey, P., Rothman, A. J., Detweiler, J. B. and Steward, W. T. (2000). Emotional states and physical health. *American Psychologist*, 55, 110–121.

Schmertz, S. K., Anderson, P. L. and Robins, D. L. (2009). The relation between self-report mindfulness and performance on tasks of sustained attention. *Journal of Psychopathology and Behavioral Assessment*, 31, 60–66.

Schmidt, N. B., Richey, J. A., Buckner, J. D. and Timpano, K. R. (2009). Attention training for generalized social anxiety disorder, *Journal of Abnormal Psychology*, 118, 5–14.

Schoeberlein, D. and Koffler, T. (2005). Garrison Institute report: Contemplation and education: A survey of programs using contemplative techniques in K–12 educational settings: A mapping report. New York: Garrison Institute. Retrieved from, http://www.garrisoninstitute.org/programs/Mapping_Report.pdf.

Semple, R. J., Lee, J. and Miller, L. F. (2006). Mindfulness-based cognitive therapy for children. In R. A. Baer, (Ed.), Mindfulness-based treatment approaches: Clinicians guide to evidence base and applications (pp. 143–166). Oxford, UK: Elsevier.

Semple, R. J., Reid, E. F. G. and Miller, L. (2005). Treating anxiety with mindfulness: An open trial of mindfulness training for anxious children. *Journal of Cognitive Psychotherapy*, 19, 379–392.

Serketich, W. J. and Dumas, J. E. (1996). The effectiveness of behavior parent training to modify antisocial behavior in children: A meta-analysis. *Behavior Therapy*, 27, 171–186.

Shonk, S. M. and Cicchetti, D. (2001). Maltreatment, competency deficits, and risk for academic and behavioral maladjustment. *Developmental Psychology*, 37, 3–17.

Simmel, C. (2007). Risk and protective factors contributing to the longitudinal psychosocial well-being of adopted foster children. *Journal of Emotional and Behavioral Disorders*, 15, 237–249.

Singh, N. N., Lancioni, G. E. Singh Joy, S. D., Winton, A. S. W., Sabaawi, M., Wahler, R. G. and Singh, J. (2007a). Adolescents with conduct disorder can be mindful of their aggressive behavior. *Journal of Emotional and Behavioral Disorders*, 15, 56–63.

Singh, N. N., Lancioni, G. E., Winton, S. W., Adkins, A. D., Wahler, R. G., Sabaawi, M. and Singh, J. (2007b). Individuals with mental illness can control their aggressive behavior through mindfulness training. *Behavior Modification*, 31, 313–328.

Singh, N. N., Lancioni, G. E., Winton, S. W., Fisher, B. C., Wahler, R. G., McAleavey, K., Singh, J. and Sabaawi, M. (2006). Mindful parenting decreases aggression, non-compliance, and self-injury in children with autism. *Journal of Emotional and Behavioral Disorders*, 14, 169–177.

Singh, N. N., Lancioni, G. E., Winton, A. S. W., Singh, J., Curtis, W. J., Wahler, R. G. and McAleavey, K. M. (2007c). Mindful parenting decreases aggression and increases social behavior in children with developmental disabilities. *Behavior Modification*, 31, 749–771.

Singh, N. N., Wahler, R. G., Adkins, A. D. and Myers, R. E. (2003). Soles of the feet: A mindfulness-based self-control intervention for aggression by an individual with mild mental retardation and mental illness. *Research in Developmental Disabilities*, 24, 158–169.

Silverman, W. K., Kurtines, W. M., Ginsburg, G. S., Weems, C. F., Lumpkin, P. W. and Carmichael, D. H. (1999). Treating anxiety disorders in children with group cognitive-behavioral therapy: A randomized clinical trial. *Journal of Consulting and Clinical Psychology*, 67, 995–1003.

Slinning, K. (2004). Foster placed children prenatally exposed to poly-substances: Attention-related problems at ages 2 and 4 1/2. *European Child and Adolescent Psychiatry*, 13, 19–27.

Spinrad, T. L., Eisenberg, N., Cumberland, A., Fabes, R. A., Valiente, C. and Shepard, S. A., et al. (2006). Relation of Emotion-Related Regulation to Children's Social Competence: A Longitudinal Study. *Emotion*, 6, 498–510.

Stein, E. (1997). Teachers' assessments of children in foster care. *Developmental Disability Bulletin*, 25(2), 1–15.

Tang, Y. Y. (2005). *Health from Brain, Wisdom from Brain*. Dalian, China: Dalian University of Technology.

Tang, Y. Y. (2007). *Multi-Intelligence and Unfolding the Full Potentials of Brain*. Dalian, China: Dalian University of Technology.

Tang, Y. Y. (2009). Exploring your brain, optimizing your life. Beijing: Science Press.

Tang, Y. Y., Ma, Y., Wang, J., Fan, Y., Feng, S., Lu, Q., Sui, D., Rothbart, M. K., Fan, M. and Posner, M. I. (2007). Short-term meditation training improves attention and self-regulation. *Proceedings of the National Academy of Sciences*, 104, 17152–17156.

Tang, Y. Y., Ma, Y., Fan, Y., Feng, H., Wang, J., Feng, S., Lu, Q., Hu, B., Lin, Y., Li, J., Zhang, Y., Wang, Y., Zhou, L. and Fan, M. (2009). Central and autonomic nervous system interaction is altered by short-term meditation. *Proceedings of the National Academy of Sciences*, 106, 8865–8870.

Taylor, J. L., Lindsay, W. R. and Willner, P. (2008). CBT for people with intellectual disabilities: emerging evidence, cognitive ability and IQ effects. *Behavioural and Cognitive Psychotherapy*, 36, 723–733.

Teasdale, J. D., Segal, Z. V. and Williams, M. G. (1995). How does cognitive therapy prevent depressive relapse and why should attentional control (mindfulness training) help? *Behaviour Research and Therapy*, 33, 25–39.

Thompson, M. and Gauntlett-Gilbert, J. (2008). Mindfulness with children and adolescents: Effective clinical application. *Clinical Child Psychology and Psychiatry*, 13, 395–407.

Trickett, P. K. and McBride-Chang, C. (1995). The developmental impact of different forms of child abuse and neglect. *Developmental Review*, 15, 311–337.

Trupin, E. W., Tarico, V. S., Low, B., Jennelka, R. and McClellan, J. (1993). Children on child protective service caseloads: Prevalence and nature of serious emotional disturbance. *Child Abuse and Neglect*, 17, 345–355.

U.S. Department of Health and Human Services. (2009). *The AFCARS Report: Preliminary FY 2008 Estimates as of October 2009*. Retrieved from, http://www. acf.hhs. gov/programs/cb/stats_research/afcars/tar/report16.htm.

U.S. General Accounting Office. (1998). Foster care agencies face challenges securing stable homes for children of substance abusers. Report to the Chairman, Committee on Finance, U.S. Senate. GAO/HEHS-98-182. Washington, DC: Government Printing Office.

U.S. General Accounting Office. (2007). Child Welfare: Additional Federal Action Could Help States Address Challenges in Providing Services to Children and Families. Testimony Before the Subcommittee on Income Security and Family Support, Committee on Ways and Means, U.S. House of Representatives. GAO-07-850T. Washington, DC: Government Printing Office.

Valentine, E. R. and Sweet, P. L. G. (1999). Meditation and attention: a comparison of the effects of concentrative and mindfulness meditation on sustained attention. *Mental Health, Religion, and Culture*, 2, 59–70.

Valiente, C., Lemery-Chalfant, K., Swanson, J. and Reiser, M. (2008). Prediction of children's academic competence from their effortful control, relationships, and classroom participation. *Journal of Educational Psychology*, 100, 67–77.

Vasey, M. W. and Ollendick, T. H. (2000). *Anxiety*. In A. J. Sameroff, M. Lewis, and S. M. Miller (Eds), Handbook of Developmental Psychopathology (pp. 511–530). New York: Klewer Academic/Plenum Publishers.

Vietin, C. and Astin, J. (2008). Effects of a minfulness-based intervention during pregnancy on prenatal stress and mood: Results of a pilot study. *Archives of Women's Mental Health*, 11, 68–74.

Vujanovic, A. A., Youngwirth, N. E., Johnson, K. A. and Zvolensky, M. J. (2009). Mindfulness-based acceptance and posttraumatic stress symptoms among trauma-exposed adults without axis I psychopathology. *Journal of Anxiety Disorders*, 23, 297–303.

Wall, R. B. (2005). Tai chi and mindfulness-based stress reduction in a Boston public middle school. *Journal of Paediatric Health Care*, 19, 230–237.

Weaver, T. L. and Clum, G. A. (1993). Early family environments and traumatic experiences associated with borderline personality disorder. *Child Abuse and Neglect*, 6, 1068–1075.

Wegner, D. and Zanakos, S. (1994). Chronic thought suppression. *Journal of Personality*, 62, 615–640.

Weinstein, N, Brown, K. W. and Ryan, R. M. (2009). A multimethod examination of the effects of mindfulness on stress attribution, coping, and emotional well-being. *Journal of Research in Personality*, 43, 374–385.

Weisz, J. R., Weiss, B., Han, S. S., Granger, D. A. and Morton, T. (1995). Effects of psychotherapy with children and adolescents revisited: A meta-analysis of treatment outcome studies. *Psychological Bulletin*, 117, 450–468.

Welch, S. L. and Fairburn, C. G. (1996). Childhood sexual and physical abuse as risk factors for the development of bulimia nervosa: A community-based case control study. *Child Abuse and Neglect*, 20, 633–642.

Wells, A. (1990). Panic disorder in association with relaxation induced anxiety: an attentional training approach to treatment. *Behavior Therapy*, 21, 273–280.

Wells, A. (2000). Emotional Disorders and Metacognition: Innovative cognitive therapy. Wiley: Chichester.

Wells, A., White, J. and Carter, K. (1997). Attention training: effects on anxiety and belief in panic and social phobia. *Clinical Psychology and Psychotherapy*, 4, 226–232.

Wentzel, K. R. and Asher, S. R. (1995). The academic lives of neglected, rejected, popular, and controversial children. *Child Development*, 66, 754–763.

Widom, C. S. and Maxfield, M. (2001). An update on the 'Cycle of violence'. National Institute of Justice: Research in Brief, February 2001.

Wodarski, J. S., Kurtz, P. D., Gaudin, J. M. and Howing, P. T. (1990). Maltreatment and the school-age child: Major academic, socioemotional, and adaptive outcomes. *Social Work*, 35, 506–513.

Zima, B. T., Bussing, R., Freeman, S., Yang, X., Belin, T. R. and Forness, S. R. (2000). Behavior problems, academic skill delays and school failure among school-aged children in foster care: Their relationship to placement characteristics. *Journal of Child and Family Studies*, 9, 87–103.

Zylowska, L., Ackerman, D. L., Yang, M. H., Futrell, J. L., Horton, N. L. and Hale, S. T., et al. (2007). Mindfulness meditation training with adults and adolescents with ADHD. *Journal of Attention Disorders*, 11, 737–746.

INDEX

A

abolition, 130

abuse, x, 22, 96, 99, 108, 116, 118, 121, 122, 123, 124, 132, 135, 137, 138, 139, 142, 143, 144, 146, 152, 153, 155, 156, 157, 158, 168, 172, 173, 174, 177, 178

academic difficulties, 155, 174, 175

academic progress, 111, 112

access, 5, 11, 13, 14, 15, 18, 21, 22, 23, 24, 25, 26, 27, 29, 31, 54, 95, 98, 106, 111, 117, 118, 120, 124, 126, 127, 129, 130, 132, 133, 134, 136, 137, 138, 146, 166, 171

accountability, 105, 113, 117, 122, 134, 137, 139, 143, 146

ACF, 2, 6, 17, 21

achievement test, 111

acid, 44

acne, 51

activism, 50

adaptability, 157

adaptation, 94, 156, 163, 166, 176

ADHD, 38, 39, 44, 50, 53, 54, 60, 63, 164, 168, 179

adjustment, 152, 153, 156, 157

Administration for Children and Families, 2, 31, 36

administrators, 7, 9, 12, 14, 15, 26, 27, 30, 81

adolescents, vii, 2, 3, 30, 31, 33, 34, 35, 45, 48, 52, 54, 55, 58, 61, 62, 98, 99, 162, 164, 165, 167, 168, 169, 171, 172, 174, 177, 178, 179

Adoptions and Safe Families Act, vii, 1

adult education, 90, 100

adulthood, 31, 39, 153

adults, 21, 37, 38, 39, 40, 42, 44, 45, 47, 48, 62, 63, 153, 162, 165, 167, 178, 179

advancement, 113

adverse effects, 22, 50, 54

adverse event, 29, 48, 61, 63

advertisements, 50

advocacy, viii, 37, 123, 139, 141, 142, 145

affective experience, 55, 158

African-American, ix, 72, 103

age, 4, 5, 6, 15, 19, 20, 22, 38, 40, 43, 47, 51, 55, 63, 69, 70, 71, 74, 75, 77, 103, 104, 109, 113, 118, 119, 128, 142, 153, 155, 157, 165, 167, 175, 178

agencies, vii, viii, ix, 1, 2, 6, 7, 9, 10, 12, 13, 14, 15, 17, 18, 19, 20, 22, 24, 25, 26, 27, 28, 29, 30, 65, 67, 82, 85, 89, 90, 92, 93, 94, 95, 96, 97, 104, 108, 109, 110, 113, 121, 129, 146, 177

aggression, 5, 106, 153, 154, 158, 162, 164, 176

aggressive behavior, 2, 172, 176

aging population, 119

AIDS, 124, 128, 130, 144

Alaska, 51

alertness, 41, 162

American Psychiatric Association, 40, 52

American Psychological Association, 50, 58, 83, 173, 174

amphetamines, 48

amygdala, 60, 164

anemia, 47

anger, 154, 155, 174

anorexia, 49

ANOVA, 71

anterior cingulate cortex, 164

anticonvulsants, viii, 37, 42, 60, 63

antidepressant medication, 45, 49, 58

antidepressant(s), viii, 20, 37, 38, 39, 41, 44, 45, 48, 49, 53, 56, 57, 58, 59, 62, 63

antipsychotic, viii, 35, 37, 39, 43, 46, 47, 50, 54, 55, 57, 58

antipsychotic drugs, viii, 35, 37, 38, 43, 46, 47, 59

antipsychotics, viii, 15, 20, 37, 39, 41, 44, 47, 50, 51, 52, 55

antisocial behavior, 153, 155, 176

anxiety, 38, 39, 45, 49, 50, 54, 58, 153, 155, 158, 161, 163, 164, 166, 168, 170, 172, 174, 176, 177, 178

anxiety disorder, 38, 39, 50, 153, 161, 168, 172, 174,
     176, 177
appetite, 48
ARC, 99
arousal, 66, 154, 155, 161, 162, 164, 166
arrhythmias, 47
Asia, 149
assessment, 3, 9, 10, 11, 12, 29, 31, 35, 45, 52, 92,
     93, 97, 107, 109, 132, 149
assessment tools, 10, 92
assets, 83
astrocytes, 59
asymptomatic, 42
ataxia, 47
attachment, 13, 93, 153, 155, 156, 161, 170, 173
attachment theory, 173
Attention Deficit Hyperactivity Disorder, 20
attentional bias, 155, 161, 168
attentional training, 178
attitudes, 90, 97, 100, 119, 123, 145
attribution, 164, 166, 178
attribution bias, 164, 166
audits, 3, 18, 19, 20, 24
authority(ies), viii, 2, 15, 78, 90, 93, 122, 128
autism, 39, 49, 55, 162, 176
autonomic nervous system, 177
avoidance, 66, 163, 172
awareness, 112, 123, 139, 143, 145, 158, 160, 161,
     162, 164, 165, 166

B

bad day, 80
balanced state, 162
barriers, 4, 12, 27, 86, 87, 90, 93, 104, 107, 109, 110,
     113, 117, 130, 137, 143, 146
base, 18, 68, 80, 87, 98, 145, 155, 165, 170, 173,
     176, 178
basic education, 133
basic research, 171
behavior of children, 168
behavior therapy, 52
behavioral disorders, 154, 169
behavioral problems, 3, 5, 21, 104, 153, 156, 166
behaviors, 9, 14, 29, 40, 121, 122, 123, 145, 154,
     156, 157, 158, 159, 163, 164, 168, 169, 174
Beijing, 148, 149, 177
beneficiaries, 127
benefits, ix, 3, 5, 13, 17, 20, 21, 22, 50, 115, 120,
     124, 126, 128, 130, 133, 137, 141, 146, 163, 169,
     171
benign, 66, 163
bias, 78, 155, 161, 165, 166, 168, 174

bipolar disorder, 53, 54, 55, 56, 57, 60, 63
bipolar illness, 57
births, 116, 119, 120, 138
bleeding, 86
blood, 47
blueprint, 99
BMI, 129, 147
borderline personality disorder, 173, 178
brain, 42, 46, 47, 50, 55, 57, 154, 164, 177
brain size, 55
breakdown, 169
breathing, 162
budget allocation, 135, 143
bulimia, 178
bulimia nervosa, 178
burnout, 66, 67, 68, 69, 71, 72, 73, 74, 77, 78, 80, 81,
     82, 83, 84
burnout scores, 77

C

campaigns, 123, 139, 141, 143, 145, 146
cancer, 163, 173
carbamazepine, 48, 53, 62, 63
cardiac arrhythmia, 47, 49
cardiovascular disease, 48, 55
care model, 145, 169
caregivers, x, 14, 15, 17, 21, 26, 29, 93, 94, 104, 105,
     106, 110, 111, 116, 118, 126, 132, 135, 138, 151,
     152, 156, 158, 159, 160, 165, 166, 167
case studies, 149, 165
case study, 99, 113
cash, 127, 128, 133, 134, 141, 144
cerebellum, 47
certificate, 108
certification, 69
cervical cancer, 130
challenges, vii, viii, ix, 2, 5, 6, 7, 8, 13, 18, 22, 24,
     28, 29, 30, 55, 56, 65, 80, 86, 88, 89, 94, 96, 100,
     107, 113, 115, 116, 121, 123, 124, 126, 146, 158,
     177
chaos, 152, 156
Chicago, 84, 113
child abuse, 3, 31, 38, 99, 122, 123, 152, 173, 177
Child Behavior Checklist, 4, 153, 167
child development, 50, 93
child labor, 118, 121
child maltreatment, 2, 81, 88, 94, 100, 141, 169, 175
child mortality, 119
child poverty, 125, 141
child protection, vii, ix, x, 65, 66, 67, 81, 82, 115,
     116, 118, 120, 121, 122, 123, 124, 125, 126, 131,

132, 133, 134, 135, 136, 138, 139, 140, 141, 142, 143, 144, 145, 146, 149

child protective services, vii, 1, 2, 33, 34

child welfare agencies, vii, viii, 1, 2, 6, 7, 9, 10, 12, 15, 17, 18, 19, 20, 22, 24, 25, 26, 28, 29, 30, 65, 67, 82, 104, 109

childcare, 83, 144

childhood, 41, 53, 55, 63, 66, 124, 129, 130, 140, 147, 149, 152, 153, 155, 156, 157, 165, 169, 170, 171, 173

childhood sexual abuse, 173

child-serving systems, vii, viii, 2, 6, 7, 85, 87, 97

China, v, vii, ix, x, 115, 116, 117, 118, 119, 120, 121, 123, 124, 125, 126, 127, 128, 129, 130, 131, 132, 133, 134, 135, 136, 137, 138, 139, 141, 142, 143, 144, 145, 146, 147, 148, 149, 162, 177

Chinese government, ix, 115, 116, 120, 123, 124, 125, 126, 127, 129, 130, 131, 134, 135, 137, 138, 140, 145

Christianity, 84

chronic illness, 163

city(ies), 68, 117, 118, 119, 127, 128, 131, 133

clarity, 80

classes, 38, 105, 106, 112

classroom, 153, 155, 178

clients, 13, 66, 68, 92, 93, 158

climate, 78, 79, 81, 82, 83, 97, 99

clinical application, 161, 162, 171, 177

clinical judgment, 9

clustering, 66

CNS, 54

coaches, 159

coastal region, 133

cognition, 60, 63, 155

cognitive ability, 166, 177

cognitive impairment, 48, 106

cognitive performance, 47, 162

cognitive process, 159

cognitive therapy, 173, 176, 177, 178

collaboration, viii, ix, 2, 5, 13, 28, 85, 94, 105, 110, 112, 113, 121, 132, 141

colleges, 110, 112

combination therapy, 46

common sense, 36

communication, 5, 17, 22, 29, 80, 81, 105, 106, 107, 123, 141, 146

community(ies), ix, x, 81, 83, 84, 85, 86, 87, 88, 93, 94, 95, 97, 107, 109, 110, 115, 116, 122, 123, 125, 128, 131, 132, 133, 134, 135, 136, 137, 139, 140, 141, 142, 143, 144, 145, 146, 152, 155, 159, 165, 169, 178

community support, 93

community-based services, 132, 140, 145

comparative analysis, 140

compassion, 67, 68, 69, 71, 74, 75, 77, 82, 83, 84

competitive markets, 79

complaints, 153, 164

complement, 6, 7

complex organizations, 79, 80, 83

complexity, 32, 79, 156

compliance, 29, 51, 86, 100, 172

compounds, 157

compulsory education, 126, 127, 130, 137, 140, 145

computer, 161

conceptual model, viii, 8, 80, 85, 88, 96, 97

conditioning, 159

conduct disorder, 2, 39, 162, 176

conference, 6

confidentiality, 22

configuration, 80

conflict, 80, 116, 138, 142, 149, 154, 164

Congress, 51, 57, 65, 142

consensus, 29, 105

consent, 5, 8, 15, 17, 35, 51, 69

consolidation, 62

construction, 129, 130

consumption, 125

control group, 44, 46, 153, 155, 161, 163, 164, 165

controlled studies, 45, 62

controversial, 178

convention, 41

conversations, 29

cooperation, 80, 107, 122, 125, 135, 142

coordination, 5, 22, 27, 83, 105, 106, 107, 112, 120, 122, 126, 134, 135, 139, 140, 142, 146

coping strategies, 163

correlation, 70, 71, 74

correlations, 74, 80

cortex, 48, 164, 175

cortisol, 163, 169, 171

cost, ix, 52, 96, 97, 109, 115, 117, 129, 130, 132, 135, 137, 141, 144, 145

cost effectiveness, 52

counseling, 67, 84, 99, 107, 122, 132, 144

covering, 143

CPU, 132, 147

cracks, 149

creativity, 90, 99

criminal behavior, 154

criminal justice system, 104

criminality, 123, 154

criminals, 126

cross-sectional study, 56

cues, 155, 161

cultural beliefs, 123

culture, 95, 97, 99, 132, 160

currency, 147
curriculum, 92, 93, 162

D

danger, 49
Darfur, 83
data collection, 69, 142
database, 20, 106, 111, 132, 141
deaths, 69
decentralization, 117
defects, 49
deficit, 53
delinquency, 153, 169
delirium, 49
delusional thinking, 43
democracy, 149
Department of Health and Human Services, 2, 6, 31, 34, 36, 61, 63, 100, 152, 156, 177
dependent variable, 71, 74
depersonalization, 66
depression, 2, 35, 38, 39, 44, 45, 49, 56, 57, 58, 59, 60, 62, 155, 158, 161, 162, 163, 164, 166, 170, 173, 175
depressive symptoms, 40, 45, 174
deprivation, 53, 139
detachment, 162
developmental psychopathology, 169
diabetes, 47, 48, 58, 61
diagnosis, 167
Diagnostic and Statistical Manual of Mental Disorders, 52
diet, 86
digestion, 154
directors, 7, 132
disability, viii, 3, 37, 127, 129, 135, 148
disaster, 127, 132
disaster assistance, 127
disaster relief, 127
discrimination, 124, 126, 138, 144
diseases, 118, 129, 130, 143
dislocation, ix, 115, 116
disorder, 20, 39, 42, 44, 45, 52, 53, 55, 63, 161, 162, 168, 174, 176, 178
dissociative disorders, 153
distortions, 155
distress, 3, 67, 68, 162, 170
District of Columbia, viii, 2
disturbances, 153
diversity, 81
dizziness, 49
doctors, 12, 45, 49, 50, 51, 52
domestic demand, 124

domestic migration, dislocation, ix, 115
domestic violence, 38, 67, 142, 158
dopamine, 46
dopaminergic, 46
dosage, 39, 46
drawing, 43
drug dependence, 5
drug withdrawal, 45
drugs, 31, 38, 39, 42, 43, 44, 45, 46, 47, 51, 52, 54, 56, 58, 106
DSM, 56
DSM-IV-TR, 40
dyslipidemia, 61
dysphoria, 52

E

East Asia, 147, 149
Eastern Europe, 99
eating disorders, 153
ecology, 35
economic boom, 116
economic development, 117, 120, 124
economic growth, ix, 115, 116, 117, 120, 124, 136
economic policy, 140
economic reform(s), 116, 117, 128, 148
economics, 26
education, 13, 23, 28, 49, 50, 51, 94, 104, 105, 106, 107, 108, 109, 110, 111, 112, 113, 116, 117, 118, 120, 122, 123, 124, 126, 127, 128, 130, 131, 132, 135, 138, 140, 141, 144, 148, 153, 176
educational experience, 104, 107
educational opportunities, 105, 109, 110, 112
educational process, 111
educational services, 13, 109
educational settings, 176
educators, 106
elementary school, 108, 109, 174
emergency, 68, 83, 108, 132, 134
emotion, 3, 154, 155, 156, 157, 158, 164, 166, 169, 173, 174, 176
emotional distress, 67
emotional exhaustion, 66, 68, 77
emotional intelligence, 165
emotional problems, 38, 107
emotional responses, 154, 156
emotionality, 41, 157, 170
empathy, 68
empirical studies, 78
employees, ix, 68, 77, 79, 80, 81, 86, 103, 129
employers, 50, 129
employment, 78, 116, 121, 130, 138
empowerment, 28, 33

endangered, 56
enforcement, 122, 134, 140, 142, 146
enrollment, ix, 103, 105, 108, 109, 112
entanglements, 51
enuresis, 47
environment(s), 21, 68, 79, 105, 121, 134, 137, 153, 155, 156, 157, 166, 178
environmental conditions, 78
epidemic, 50, 53, 63
epilepsy, 53, 57
equity, 124, 138
ethics, 51
ethnicity, 19
everyday life, 172
evidence, viii, x, 5, 6, 7, 11, 13, 18, 21, 30, 32, 35, 36, 38, 40, 42, 43, 44, 45, 50, 68, 80, 81, 83, 85, 86, 87, 88, 90, 92, 93, 94, 95, 96, 97, 98, 99, 100, 140, 142, 144, 146, 151, 152, 156, 158, 159, 166, 167, 170, 172, 176, 177
evidence-based policy, 142, 146
evidence-based program, 100
execution, 67
executive function, 153, 154, 155, 157, 166, 168, 175
executive functioning, 153, 155, 166
executive functions, 168, 175
exercise, 52, 81, 161
expenditures, 100, 123, 134
experiences, 152, 161, 163
expertise, viii, 2, 8, 12, 14, 15, 25, 26, 29, 96
exploitation, x, 116, 118, 119, 121, 122, 123, 124, 132, 137, 138, 139, 143, 144, 146
exploration, 166
exposure, 47, 55, 58, 66, 67, 68, 69, 77, 81, 106, 158, 167, 173
expulsion, 112
externalizing behavior, 5, 153, 154, 157, 164, 168, 174
externalizing disorders, 169

family support, 121, 122, 126, 131, 135, 136, 139, 140, 144, 145, 152, 171
family system, 3, 93
family therapy, 69
family violence, 67, 82, 142, 152
farmers, 124
fat, 46, 47
fatty acids, 53
fear, 154
federal government, viii, 6, 37, 52
feelings, 66, 154
fertility, 119, 148
fibromyalgia, 163, 171, 172, 173
fidelity, 89, 90, 92, 93, 94, 95, 96, 97, 99, 163
financial, 25, 29, 49, 50, 61, 79, 95, 109, 117, 127, 134, 139, 141, 143, 145, 146
financial resources, 25, 134
financial support, 95
fish, 44
flexibility, 81, 99, 155, 166
flight, 80, 154
fluctuations, 49
fluoxetine, 45, 46, 49, 62
fluvoxamine, 45, 48, 61
folic acid, 130
food, 58, 86, 126, 127, 148
Food and Drug Administration (FDA), 20, 38, 42, 44, 45, 47, 48, 49, 50, 58, 60, 62, 63
force, 81
formal sector, 129
foster youth, 104, 105, 106, 107, 109, 110, 111, 112, 113
foundations, 7
fraud, 52
freedom, 78
Freud, 81
fruits, 86
funding, viii, 10, 25, 28, 30, 85, 93, 95, 96, 109, 110, 112, 123, 127, 128, 152
funds, 89, 94, 108, 109, 128, 129, 137, 146

F

Facebook, 79
fairness, 80, 81
false positive, 41
families, vii, ix, 4, 22, 23, 29, 30, 33, 41, 93, 94, 96, 111, 115, 116, 117, 118, 119, 120, 122, 124, 126, 127, 128, 130, 131, 132, 133, 134, 135, 138, 141, 144, 145, 146, 157, 158, 160, 166, 168, 175
family environment, 178
family members, ix, 40, 115, 116
family planning, 119, 138

G

GDP, 117, 147
gender equality, 120
General Accounting Office (GAO), viii, 6, 32, 37, 38, 51, 52, 65, 82, 152, 153, 177, 178
general education, 107
Generalized Anxiety Disorder, 155, 161, 168, 174
genes, 40
genetic predisposition, 40
Georgia, 37
Germany, 98

gestation, 49
Gini coefficients, 120
glial cells, 46
good behavior, 123
goose, 54
governance, 135, 139, 147
government procurement, 133, 137
governments, 117, 121, 123, 126, 130
grades, 109, 111, 153
grants, 30, 51
group therapy, 87
growth, 46, 48, 82, 119, 124, 135
growth hormone, 48
Guangzhou, 133
guardian, 107, 109, 121, 157
guidance, 6, 7, 14, 27, 30, 32, 129, 137
guidelines, 6, 7, 8, 9, 10, 12, 13, 14, 20, 21, 22, 23,
    24, 25, 26, 27, 28, 29, 33, 34, 35, 49, 51, 56, 136,
    141, 142, 144, 145, 159
guilty, 52

H

hallucinations, 43
harmony, 162
hazards, viii, 37
headache, 49
Health and Human Services, 156, 177
health care, 2, 4, 5, 6, 7, 9, 11, 13, 17, 18, 24, 25, 27,
    28, 29, 30, 31, 33, 35, 71, 75, 86, 87, 98, 117,
    124, 129, 132, 137, 171
health services, vii, viii, 1, 2, 3, 4, 5, 6, 8, 13, 14, 21,
    25, 27, 30, 32, 33, 55, 98, 108, 128, 129, 173
health status, 31, 35, 169
heart attack, 48, 108
heart disease, 163
heart rate, 58
height, 48, 55, 63
hepatitis, 48, 130
hepatitis a, 48
HHS, 6, 32, 82
high school, 104, 105, 109, 111, 112, 113
high-risk populations, 167
Hispanics, 71
history, vii, ix, 1, 4, 13, 38, 58, 68, 103, 106, 111,
    175
HIV, 118, 124, 125, 128, 132, 135, 138, 145, 146
HIV/AIDS, 118, 124, 125, 128, 132, 135, 138, 145,
    146
homelessness, 152
homeostasis, 53
homes, 54, 105, 160, 177
homework, 105

Hops, 158, 173
host, 29, 152, 154, 156, 158, 161
House, 53, 148, 178
House of Representatives, 178
housing, 127
human, 25, 28, 29, 57, 62, 81, 89, 119, 123, 125,
    133, 136, 139, 141, 143
human development, 119
human resources, 28, 136, 139, 141, 143
hygiene, 86, 100
hyperactivity, 53, 106, 154, 155
hyperandrogenism, 57
hypochondriasis, 161, 174
hypospadias, 49
hypothesis, 42, 43, 45, 80

I

ideal, 135
ideal forms, 135
identification, 13, 41, 99, 122, 132, 141
identity, 79
illusion, 53
images, 46
immune response, 47
immunization, 108, 129
impacts, 164
improvements, 81, 92, 112, 116, 127, 162, 164
impulses, 154, 156
impulsivity, 5, 48, 155, 158, 168, 171
in vivo, 159
inattention, 155
incarceration, 112, 159, 169
incidence, 86, 119
income, 116, 117, 119, 120, 127, 132, 138
income inequality, 120
Independence, 159, 171
independent living, 131
independent variable, 74, 76
individual character, 79
individual characteristics, 79
individual differences, 97
individualization, x, 151
individuals, 9, 42, 43, 46, 49, 68, 69, 70, 73, 80, 90,
    104, 162, 163, 164, 168
industry, 49, 50, 51, 57, 79
inequality, 148, 149
infants, 49, 129
inflammation, 58
information processing, 161
informed consent, 15, 17, 20, 23, 51, 52, 69
infrastructure, 81, 89
inhibition, 48, 168

injury(ies), 121, 123, 127, 129, 168, 176
inoculation, 81
insomnia, 38, 48, 49
Institute of Justice, 178
institutions, 119, 123, 129, 131, 133, 135, 136, 149
integration, 146
intellectual capital, 79, 83
intellectual disabilities, 130, 158, 177
intelligence, 165
interdependence, 79
interference, 164, 174
internalizing, 153, 155, 157
international standards, 125, 140, 142
intervention, viii, x, 5, 12, 21, 27, 30, 43, 59, 65, 69,
    77, 94, 99, 105, 106, 107, 108, 109, 111, 151,
    152, 153, 156, 158, 159, 160, 162, 163, 164, 168,
    170, 174, 175, 176, 178
intimacy, 66
intrinsic motivation, 176
intrusions, 170
investment(s), 112, 117, 125
invitation to participate, 69
Iraq, 41
irritability, 41, 49
isolation, 8, 30, 110
issues, vii, ix, x, 12, 13, 23, 31, 62, 63, 80, 93, 97,
    104, 108, 110, 112, 115, 120, 122, 123, 124, 126,
    135, 141, 145, 149, 151, 152, 171, 172

J

job satisfaction, 77
junior high school, 108
jurisdiction, 112
justification, 52
juvenile justice, viii, 28, 85, 86, 87, 88, 97, 113, 142

K

kidney, 47, 53
kindergarten, ix, 103, 173
kinship, 3, 4, 15, 126, 135, 136, 140, 160, 169

L

labeling, 41, 164, 170
lack of control, 163
lack of personal accomplishment, 77
latency, 53
later life, 40
laws, ix, 115, 121, 122, 123, 125, 126, 127, 139, 140,
    141, 142, 143

laws and regulations, 140
lawyers, 143
LEA, 108, 109
lead, 50, 110, 139, 166
leadership, viii, 2, 29, 30, 79, 88, 89, 90, 92, 95, 96
Leahy, 90, 100
learning, viii, 63, 85, 88, 89, 90, 91, 92, 93, 95, 96,
    105, 106, 107, 159, 174
legislation, vii, 1, 3, 6, 7, 108, 109, 110, 112, 142
lending, 164
lethargy, 49, 86
liberty, 10
licensure board rosters, viii, 65
life cycle, 81
light, ix, 43, 44, 63, 115, 121, 124, 144
literacy, 21, 29, 33
lithium, 43, 47, 53, 55, 57, 60, 61
living arrangements, 131
local community, 14, 26, 123
local government, 117, 127, 128, 130, 134
longitudinal study, 58
loss of libido, 48

M

magnitude, 45
mainstream society, 131
major depression, 38, 39, 53, 54, 175
major depressive disorder, 55
majority, 10, 12, 15, 43, 103, 104, 116, 136, 152, 164
malaise, 86
maltreatment, x, 32, 36, 66, 104, 121, 151, 152, 153,
    155, 169, 170, 175
man, 49, 161, 162
management, 12, 13, 21, 35, 81, 84, 93, 99, 111, 122,
    129, 132, 136, 137, 141, 142, 143, 144, 154, 159,
    160, 172, 174
mania, 40, 42, 43, 48, 49, 53, 57, 58, 62, 63
manic, 41, 43, 53, 57, 59, 61
manic-depressive psychosis, 61
mapping, 141, 176
market economy, 117
marketing, 51
marketplace, 78, 79, 80
marriage, 69
Maryland, 170
materials, 51, 94, 137
matter, 159
measurement, 4, 84, 96, 100, 167
media, 121
Medicaid, viii, 2, 3, 4, 5, 6, 10, 12, 14, 18, 19, 20, 22,
    24, 25, 26, 27, 28, 29, 33, 34, 36, 38, 39, 49, 51,
    52, 58, 59, 61

medical, 5, 7, 13, 14, 17, 22, 23, 25, 26, 32, 44, 50, 51, 58, 98, 123, 127, 128, 129, 130, 133, 134, 137, 141, 143, 145, 163
medical assistance, 137
medication, vii, 1, 3, 5, 6, 7, 12, 13, 15, 18, 19, 20, 24, 25, 27, 28, 30, 31, 34, 35, 36, 38, 46, 47, 49, 51, 57, 58, 61, 62, 63
medicine, 51, 55, 61
membership, viii, 65, 69, 78
memorandums of understanding, 125
memory, 44, 49, 62, 63
memory formation, 44
mental disorder, 21, 33, 34, 38, 50
mental health needs, vii, viii, 1, 2, 7, 9, 13, 21, 25, 29, 32, 33, 172
mental health professionals, 21, 25
mental illness, viii, 4, 34, 37, 38, 53, 57, 152, 162, 176
mental retardation, 28, 162, 176
mentorship, 89
meta-analysis, 43, 45, 58, 60, 62, 82, 104, 163, 171, 173, 174, 176, 178
metabolic syndrome, 48
methodology, 98, 162, 163, 167
methylphenidate, 48, 63
Mexico, 68
Miami, 175
migrant population, 118
migrants, 117, 118, 129, 137
migration, ix, 115, 116, 118, 125, 126, 136
Ministry of Education, 130, 147, 148
mission, 6, 24, 29, 78, 79, 81, 103
Missouri, 21
models, viii, x, 60, 70, 71, 78, 85, 96, 115, 116, 128, 133, 139, 142, 143, 144, 145, 162
modification, 161, 168
modifications, 92, 94
modules, 145
monitoring, 160, 163, 164
mood disorder, 56, 62
mood stabilizers, viii, 20, 37, 39, 41, 51, 59
morale, 80
morbidity, 22, 53, 118, 173
mortality, 116, 118, 120, 173
mortality rate, 116, 120
motivation, 90, 176
motor tic, 48
movement disorders, 47
MSW, 52
mucous membrane, 86
multidimensional, 122
multivariate, 70
muscle spasms, 49

Myanmar, 125, 142

N

narratives, 79, 92, 93
National Academy of Sciences, 177
National Child Traumatic Stress Network, ix, 83, 85, 89, 98
National Institute of Mental Health, 27, 34, 45
National Institutes of Health, 34
national policy, 141
National Survey, 38
natural disaster(s), ix, 115, 116, 125
nausea, 47, 49
negative attitudes, 123
negative consequences, 6, 157
negative effects, 118
negative emotions, 163
negative outcomes, 117, 123
negativity, 154
neglect, x, 2, 3, 4, 31, 38, 52, 96, 108, 116, 121, 122, 123, 124, 132, 135, 138, 139, 144, 146, 152, 153, 155, 156, 157, 177
negotiating, 118
nephropathy, 59, 60
nervous system, 177
neural network(s), 154
neurobiology, x, 151, 171, 175
neurogenesis, 63
neuroleptic drugs, 47
neuroleptics, 46
neurotransmitter, 46
neutral, 161, 162, 164
New England, 33, 51, 54, 57
New Zealand, 62, 171
No Child Left Behind, 109
nonprofit organizations, 133, 137
North America, 35, 62, 97
NPS, 107
nurses, 25, 26, 83
nursing, 129
nutrition, 58, 118, 127, 148, 149

O

obesity, 163
obsessive-compulsive disorder, 60
obstacles, x, 151, 152, 167
offenders, 142, 169
olanzapine, 47, 55, 61, 63
old age, 119
omega-3, 44

openness, viii, 85, 90
operant conditioning, 159
opportunities, ix, 77, 80, 81, 86, 104, 147
Oppositional Defiant Disorder, 20
organizational culture, 27, 81, 95
outpatient(s), 2, 4, 5, 23, 34, 35, 54, 60, 67, 69, 71, 73, 74, 169
outreach, 131, 133, 140
outsourcing, 133
ovaries, 57
overlap, 41, 138
oversight, vii, viii, 1, 2, 5, 6, 7, 8, 14, 25, 28, 29, 30, 31, 32, 34, 35, 112
overtime, 110

P

Pacific, 147, 149
pain, 163, 172
pancreatitis, 48
panic disorder, 5, 161
panic symptoms, 163
paradigm shift, 93
parallel, 121, 124, 127, 136
parental care, 14, 118, 123, 126, 131, 135, 138, 145
parental consent, 109
parental involvement, 93
parenthood, 152
parenting, x, 32, 38, 118, 123, 140, 151, 159, 165, 166, 171, 176
parents, vii, 1, 14, 15, 21, 22, 23, 29, 38, 39, 40, 49, 51, 52, 66, 93, 107, 118, 119, 121, 125, 126, 128, 132, 137, 138, 144, 156, 159, 162, 166, 169, 170, 175
parietal cortex, 58
parietal lobe, 46
parole, 159
participants, viii, 46, 65, 69, 71, 91, 92, 104, 113, 128, 161, 163, 164, 165
pathology, x, 151
pathways, 79, 173
penalties, 126
per capita income, 127
performance, 154, 164, 170, 176
permission, 3
perpetrators, 84
personal accomplishment, 66
personal communication, 52
personality, 62, 153, 154, 173, 175, 178
personality disorder, 153, 154, 173, 178
pharmaceutical(s), 42, 49, 50, 51
pharmacological treatment, 14, 24
pharmacotherapy, 43

phenotype, 58
phobia, 161, 168, 178
photographs, 3
physical abuse, 3, 155, 178
physical health, 89, 163, 176
physicians, 39, 50, 51, 52
Physiological, 154
physiological arousal, 164
pilot study, 61, 171, 173, 178
placebo, 42, 44, 45, 53, 55, 56, 61, 62
plasticity, 170
polarity, 55, 58
police, 132
policy, viii, x, 2, 3, 6, 7, 9, 17, 25, 29, 30, 31, 32, 34, 35, 36, 55, 77, 81, 89, 98, 106, 107, 112, 115, 119, 121, 123, 124, 125, 126, 127, 128, 130, 133, 134, 135, 137, 139, 140, 141, 142, 143, 144, 146, 148, 159
policymakers, 81, 87, 97, 104, 110
population, 2, 5, 8, 10, 18, 21, 24, 25, 28, 29, 38, 40, 41, 46, 50, 57, 62, 67, 88, 93, 104, 105, 107, 111, 112, 116, 117, 118, 119, 120, 127, 128, 136, 138, 143, 148, 149, 152, 153, 156, 158, 165, 166
population group, 116, 119, 120
portability, 129
positive mental health, 11
positive reinforcement, 160
positive relationship, 67
post traumatic stress disorder, 168
posttraumatic stress, 173, 178
post-traumatic stress disorder, 5
poverty, ix, 112, 115, 116, 117, 120, 124, 127, 128, 133, 138, 139, 141, 148, 149, 152
poverty alleviation, 116, 124
poverty line, 116, 117, 127, 133
poverty reduction, 116, 124, 138, 149
predictor variables, 70, 71, 74
prefrontal cortex, 164, 175
pregnancy, 49, 55, 56, 62, 129, 178
prejudice, 148
preparedness, 153
preschool, 98, 106, 112, 130, 155, 175
preschool children, 98
preschoolers, 62, 157, 171
President, 87, 100
prevalence rate, 119
prevention, viii, x, 21, 53, 61, 65, 99, 106, 109, 118, 122, 126, 128, 129, 132, 135, 138, 139, 141, 142, 151, 167
primary caregivers, 156
primary school, 117, 130
principles, 31, 93, 158, 159, 162
prioritizing, 165

private sector, 137
probability, 24, 39, 78
problem behavior, 35, 155, 157, 159, 168, 170, 174
problem behaviors, 35, 155, 157, 168, 174
problem-solving, 158
professional development, 81
professionals, vii, viii, 11, 26, 28, 65, 66, 67, 68, 69, 71, 72, 73, 75, 77, 78, 80, 81, 83, 84, 107, 136, 142, 145, 159
prognosis, 43
programming, 81, 139, 142
project, ix, 85, 94, 118
prosocial behavior, 159
protection, ix, x, 14, 29, 67, 115, 116, 118, 120, 121, 122, 123, 124, 125, 126, 127, 128, 129, 130, 131, 132, 133, 134, 135, 136, 137, 138, 139, 140, 141, 142, 143, 144, 145, 146, 147, 149
protective factors, x, 68, 151, 156, 166, 176
Prozac, 45, 46, 49
psoriasis, 163
psychiatric disorders, 34, 50, 155
psychiatrist, 11, 13, 25, 39, 51
psychiatry, 7, 14, 27, 51, 53, 56, 57, 60, 88, 100
psychological development, 118, 153
psychological distress, 21, 66, 67, 82, 170
psychological well-being, 169
psychology, 69, 88, 99, 101, 175
psychopathology, 169, 170, 178
psychopharmacological treatments, 14
psychopharmacology, 3, 8, 13, 15, 18, 62
psychosis, 39, 41, 43, 48, 53, 59, 60, 62
psychosocial functioning, 24, 33, 173
psychosocial interventions, 26, 168
psychosocial support, 122, 126, 132, 143, 145
psychotherapy, 5, 14, 43, 52, 67, 77, 100, 178
psychotic symptoms, 43
psychotropic drugs, 6, 38, 51
psychotropic medications, 3, 5, 6, 13, 15, 18, 20, 21, 24, 25, 26, 32, 35, 45, 51, 54, 101
PTSD, 5, 38, 41, 67, 98, 158, 166, 170
puberty, 48
public awareness, 123, 139, 140, 141, 143, 145
public financing, 135
public health, 14, 25, 26, 27, 28, 29, 118, 120, 127, 133, 140, 152
public officials, 117, 146
public schools, 118, 130
public sector, 80, 123, 137
public service, 97, 118, 134, 138, 140, 144
publishing, 39
pulmonary hypertension, 49, 54
punishment, 123

Q

quality improvement, 8, 25, 91, 92, 93
quality of life, x, 67, 77, 84, 116, 151, 164
questioning, 40, 104
questionnaire, 62

R

race, 19, 69, 70, 71, 74, 75, 76, 77
racing, 161
random assignment, 42, 46
rating scale, 9, 10
reactions, 13, 156
reactivity, 153
reading, ix, 50, 103, 104, 111
real time, 18, 95
reality, 45
reception, 154
recognition, 21, 24
recommendations, 10, 12, 13, 20, 32, 49
reconstruction, 127
recovery, 122
recurrence, 60
reform(s), x, 33, 56, 98, 113, 115, 117, 141, 142, 146, 147, 149
regression, 70, 71, 74, 76
regression equation, 70, 71
regression model, 70, 71, 74
regulations, 122, 136, 142, 143
regulatory framework, 122, 137
rehabilitation, 126, 130, 131, 137, 142, 156
reinforcement, 160
rejection, 166
relapses, 45, 46
relatives, 4, 40, 43, 118, 157, 170
relaxation, 159, 161, 162, 164, 178
relevance, 43, 96, 171
relief, 68, 131
religion, 67, 68
remediation, 156
remission, 42, 44, 62
replication, x, 115, 132, 144
requirements, 15, 25, 89, 112, 126, 137, 152, 159
researchers, 14, 26, 40, 67, 78, 80, 154, 160, 167
Residential, 83
residuals, 74
resilience, x, 80, 121, 151, 152, 166, 167, 169, 170
resolution, 124
resource allocation, 68

resources, vii, viii, 2, 8, 14, 27, 28, 29, 35, 68, 78, 79, 87, 88, 90, 92, 94, 95, 100, 106, 107, 110, 111, 117, 121, 134, 147, 148, 149, 166
response, 6, 7, 13, 21, 24, 39, 46, 48, 53, 61, 66, 69, 122, 124, 132, 135, 141, 154, 156, 164, 169
restrictions, 118
restructuring, 117, 129
retardation, 162, 176
retention rate, 169
rights, 108, 109, 118, 121, 125, 126, 138, 139, 145, 146
risk factors, 21, 121, 122, 139, 166, 167, 178
risks, ix, 3, 13, 20, 21, 22, 50, 115, 116, 120, 121, 122, 124, 135, 136, 137, 138, 139
risperidone, 61
rodents, 42
role playing, 90
root(s), 30, 31, 71, 74, 137, 160
routes, 118
routines, 159
rule of law, 120, 122
rules, 3, 78, 129, 135, 143
rural areas, 14, 27, 117, 118, 120, 121, 124, 127, 128, 130, 132, 133, 134, 137, 138, 144
rural counties, 127, 130
rural population, 116, 118, 128
rural women, 130

S

safety, vii, 1, 3, 6, 19, 25, 29, 55, 58, 65, 66, 80, 84, 104, 135, 159
SAMHSA, 172
sample survey, 148
schistosomiasis, 130
schizophrenia, 39, 41, 59, 60
school, ix, 5, 14, 26, 44, 48, 63, 69, 74, 103, 104, 105, 106, 107, 108, 109, 110, 111, 112, 113, 114, 117, 118, 123, 126, 130, 137, 145, 153, 154, 156, 157, 159, 165, 168, 169, 174, 178, 179
school performance, 44, 48, 157
schooling, 105, 110, 112
science, viii, 85, 89, 97, 100, 167
scope, 7, 24, 139, 140
secondary education, 116, 130
security, 118, 122, 126, 127, 136
seizure, 42, 60
selective serotonin reuptake inhibitor, 48, 55, 59, 61, 62
self-awareness, 158, 165, 166
self-control, 176
self-monitoring, 154
self-mutilation, 46
self-reflection, 165
self-regulation, x, 151, 153, 154, 155, 156, 157, 164, 166, 172, 175, 177
self-report data, 67
self-study, 89
semi-structured interviews, 9, 10
Senate, 51, 52, 57, 58, 61, 177
sensations, 49, 160
senses, 160
sensitivity, 42
sensitization, 60
September 11, 68, 84
serotonin, 54, 55
sertraline, 45, 59, 170
service provider, 123, 133
service quality, 80
sex, 119
sexual abuse, 4, 84, 98, 100, 121, 155, 158, 168, 172, 173, 174
sexual violence, 119
shelter, 131, 136, 144, 156
showing, 111, 132, 136
siblings, 107, 118
side effects, 13, 17, 19, 47, 51, 55, 59
simulation, 94
skewness, 74
skin, 86
sleep disorders, 39, 48
social attitudes, 119, 139, 145, 161, 176
social behavior, 122, 123, 140, 162, 176
social benefits, 118, 133, 137
social competence, 153, 170, 173
social consequences, 119, 124
social desirability, 78
social development, 48, 176
social exclusion, 120, 122, 138, 139
social inequalities, 138
social learning, 159
social norms, 119, 123
social phobia, 161, 168, 178
social protection programs, ix, 115, 118, 135
social security, 119, 124, 129
Social Security, 49, 130
social services, ix, 28, 115, 117, 118, 121, 122, 123, 124, 132, 133, 134, 136, 137, 138, 144, 146, 152
social skills, 106, 165, 173, 174
social support, 144
social welfare, ix, x, 115, 116, 117, 118, 120, 121, 122, 124, 131, 133, 134, 135, 136, 137, 138, 141, 145
social workers, 21, 67, 69, 82, 106, 107, 110, 111, 122, 123, 132, 133, 135, 136, 141, 142, 143, 146
societal cost, 61

society, 57, 123, 124, 127

sociology, 78

software, 70, 71

solidarity, 79

special education, ix, 103, 104, 105, 106, 107, 111, 112, 113, 153

specialists, 12, 14, 27, 29, 81

species, 48

speech, 47

spending, 52, 56, 134

spirituality, 67, 83, 84, 174

stability, 18, 24, 55, 104, 108, 109, 120, 158, 159, 165, 166

stabilizers, viii, 20, 37, 39, 41, 51, 59

staff development, 99

staffing, 25, 28

stakeholder groups, 14, 26, 89

stakeholders, 5, 7, 9, 13, 15, 17, 23, 25, 27, 28, 88, 96, 97

standard deviation, 71

standard error, 74, 76

standard of living, 128

state-owned enterprises, 129

states, viii, 6, 7, 10, 15, 18, 19, 20, 22, 26, 28, 29, 32, 35, 38, 51, 52, 65, 109, 111, 121, 128, 152, 154, 159, 176

statistics, 31, 138, 148

Stevens-Johnson syndrome, 48, 54

stigma, 124, 138, 144

stimulant, 44, 48, 55

stimulus, 154, 155, 161

strategic planning, 141

stress, vii, x, 33, 44, 65, 66, 67, 68, 69, 77, 80, 81, 82, 83, 84, 151, 152, 155, 157, 161, 163, 165, 166, 168, 169, 171, 172, 173, 174, 178

stress response, 68

stressful events, 156

stressors, 80, 82, 155, 156, 158, 166

structural barriers, 87

structure, 27, 87, 143, 159

style, 92, 170

subgroups, 68, 111

subsidy, 128, 136, 141, 144

subsistence, 127, 130

substance abuse, 82, 99, 152, 154, 177

substance use, 10, 68

suicidal ideation, 46, 48, 153, 158

suicide, 46, 51, 175

supervision, viii, 13, 80, 82, 83, 85, 88, 89, 90, 91, 92, 93, 95, 118, 159

supervisor(s), ix, 15, 67, 78, 80, 81, 82, 86, 89, 92, 94, 95

supplementation, 44, 58

support services, 119, 122, 131, 152

suppression, 42, 48, 163, 170, 178

surveillance, 53, 148

survey, 152, 176

survival, 116, 138, 145

survivors, 158, 169

suspensions, 153

sustainability, 94, 95, 97, 135, 145

Switzerland, 86, 150

symptoms, 23, 33, 38, 40, 41, 42, 43, 44, 45, 46, 47, 49, 54, 56, 60, 62, 66, 67, 68, 69, 86, 98, 155, 158, 161, 163, 164, 166, 170, 173, 174, 175, 178

syndrome, 48, 57

synergistic effect, 79

synthesis, 59, 77, 82, 99

systemic change, 90, 111

T

talk therapy, 41

Tamhane test, 72, 73

tar, 36, 63, 177

tardive dyskinesia, 47, 60

target, 13, 21, 130, 162

Task Force, 7, 9, 12, 14, 25, 27, 28, 31, 32, 133, 148

teachers, 105, 107, 122, 130, 132, 135, 142, 145, 153, 155, 159, 175

teams, 79, 91, 95, 111

technical assistance, 6, 139, 140, 141, 142, 145

techniques, 90, 94, 161, 165, 166, 176

technology(ies), 94, 119

tension(s), 96, 107, 124, 161

terminals, 131

terrorism, 158

terrorist attack, 68

test scores, 104, 111, 112, 153

textbook, 130

therapeutic agents, 159

therapeutic relationship, 158

therapist, 82, 84, 93, 94

therapy, 26, 61, 62, 87, 94, 100, 158, 163, 168, 169, 170, 172, 173, 174, 176, 177, 178

thoughts, 154, 158, 160, 161, 162, 163, 164

threats, 74, 86

thyroid, 47

tissue, 46, 55

Title I, 109

trafficking, 118, 119, 121, 125, 126, 137, 138, 142, 144, 146

trainees, 82, 92, 95

training programs, 88, 163, 173

trajectory, 21, 112, 159

transformation(s), 33, 71, 74

transition to adulthood, 21
transmission, 128, 141
transparency, 5, 137
transplantation, 56
transport, 108
transportation, 5, 108, 109, 118
trauma, v, vii, 1, 2, 4, 13, 29, 41, 66, 67, 68, 69, 77,
    81, 82, 83, 84, 85, 91, 92, 93, 94, 95, 97, 98, 99,
    105, 132, 155, 158, 166, 169, 170, 171, 178
traumatic experiences, 18, 81, 178
treaties, 125
treatment methods, 162
tremor, 49
trial, 44, 53, 54, 55, 58, 61, 98, 142, 168, 169, 170,
    171, 173, 176, 177
troubleshooting, 110
tuberculosis, 130
tuition, 130
turnover, 83, 89, 90, 95, 96, 97, 99
tutoring, 106, 107, 108, 109

U

UK, 54, 176
unemployment insurance, 118, 129
uniform, 18
uninsured, 127
United Nations (UN), 116, 121, 125, 147, 148, 149
United States (US), viii, 1, 30, 31, 32, 35, 37, 58, 65,
    103, 152, 165
United, viii, 1, 30, 32, 35, 37, 58, 65, 103, 121, 125,
    147, 149, 152, 165
universal access, 120, 127, 130, 133
urban areas, 4, 118, 119, 127, 128, 130, 137, 144
urban population, 118, 129
urban, 4, 69, 70, 71, 74, 75, 117, 118, 119, 127, 128,
    129, 130, 131, 133, 137, 140, 141, 144
urbanization, ix, 115, 116, 118, 136
urethra, 49

V

vaccinations, 130
vaccine, 118
validation, 62, 82, 84
variables, 62, 68, 70, 71, 74, 76, 78, 157
variations, 32, 67, 68, 134
vein, 136
venlafaxine, 59
victimization, 154
victims, 2, 138, 142, 153

Vietnam, 125, 142
violence, x, 66, 77, 116, 118, 119, 121, 122, 123,
    124, 125, 132, 138, 139, 142, 143, 144, 145, 146,
    149, 152, 158, 178
vision, 28, 93, 140, 141
vitamin C, 86
vitamin C deficiency, 86
vocational training, 130, 131, 132, 137
vomiting, 47
vulnerability, vii, 117, 120, 121, 122, 124, 126, 128,
    136, 139, 141, 144

W

waiver, 69
war, 62, 108, 148
Washington, 30, 31, 32, 51, 52, 83, 100, 113, 148,
    149, 168, 171, 173, 174, 177, 178
web, 48, 51, 91
weight gain, 19, 47, 48, 54, 58, 61
welfare law, 140
welfare system, vii, ix, 2, 3, 4, 5, 8, 13, 14, 23, 24,
    26, 61, 81, 104, 107, 113, 115, 120, 121, 132,
    134, 136, 139, 140, 141, 148, 149, 152
well-being, vii, x, 1, 3, 6, 29, 36, 65, 118, 123, 125,
    128, 151, 152, 163, 165, 166, 169, 176, 178
withdrawal, 49, 54, 59, 66
work activities, 91
workers, viii, 12, 14, 15, 18, 26, 28, 51, 65, 66, 67,
    68, 69, 70, 71, 73, 74, 77, 78, 79, 80, 81, 82, 83,
    84, 106, 107, 111, 122, 129, 132, 133, 135, 136,
    138, 141, 142, 143, 145, 146, 149, 172
workforce, 77, 81, 82
workplace, 65, 68, 79, 80, 84
World Bank, 116, 117, 124, 127, 128, 133, 148, 149
World Health Organization (WHO), 128, 147, 150

Y

young adults, 31, 43
young people, 149
young women, 47, 119
youth transition, 23, 31

Z

Zoloft, 45

DATE DUE	RETURNED